Prehospital & Emergency
Ultrasound
Logbook & Guide

Dr T E Mallinson

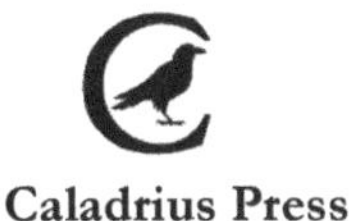

Caladrius Press

Published by
Caladrius Press
Office 140238
PO Box 6945
London
England
W1A 6US

1st Edition
3

ISBN: 978-1-917521-06-2

Contents

Preface

This small text seeks to provide an ultrasound logbook for use at the bedside. It aims to meet the needs of prehospital and emergency medicine clinicians seeking to develop their capabilities in point of care ultrasound and allow the gathering of evidence to support their progression in relation to post-graduate training and development in relation to the concept of entrustment.

The signature library on the following page allows you to keep a record of those who have assessed or supervised your imaging, while the following logs allow you to record numbers of scans undertaken in the classroom (Supervised Simulated Practice), while being mentored in practice (Supervised Clinical Practice) and when developing your skills as an autonomous clinician (Independent Clinical Practice).

While primarily a logbook, **Quick Guides** have also been included to refresh the clinician's memory of a specific scanning protocol, and to act as a handy revision tool.

The following scanning protocols and techniques are included:
- Extended Focused Assessment with Sonography in Trauma (eFAST)
- Aorta (AAA),
- Vascular Access,
- Echo in Life Support,
- Inferior Vena Cava (IVC),
- Optic Nerve Sheath Diameter (ONSD),
- Nerve Block,
- Rapid Ultrasound for Shock & Hypotension (RUSH),

and the
- Rapid DVT Protocol.

The logbook is designed to allow documentation of scan acquisitions in numbers which meet the standards set out by the Royal College of Emergency Medicine and the author is grateful for the hard work of that College in improving standards for point of care education and competency demonstration.

Dr T E Mallinson
September 2024

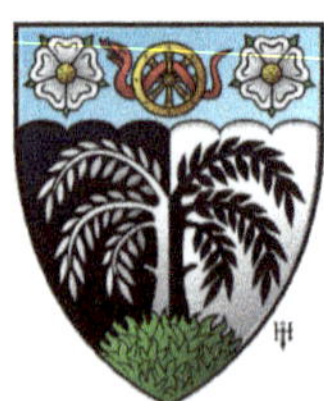

<u>Signature Library</u>

NAME / SIGNATURE / INITIALS / STAMP	ROLE / QUALIFICATIONS
NAME / SIGNATURE / INITIALS / STAMP	ROLE / QUALIFICATIONS

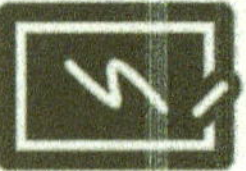

LOG
Supervised Simulated Practice
Preparing for Ultrasound in Practice

	eFAST		AAA (Aorta)		Vascular Access		Echo in Life Support	
	Date	Sign	Date	Sign	Date	Sign	Date	Sign
1								
2								
3								
4								
5								
6								
7								
8								
9								
10								
11								
12								
13								
14								
15								
16								
17								
18								
19								
20								
21								
22								
23								
24								
25								
26								
27								
28								
29								
30								

LOG
Supervised Simulated Practice
Preparing for Ultrasound in Practice

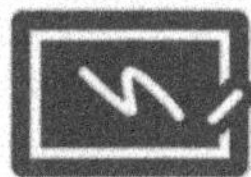

IVC (Vena Cava) Measurement		ICP ONSD (Optic Nerve)		Nerve Block		RUSH		Rapid DVT		
Date	Sign	Date	Sign	Date	Sign	Date	Sign	Date	Sign	1
										2
										3
										4
										5
										6
										7
										8
										9
										10
										11
										12
										13
										14
										15
										16
										17
										18
										19
										20
										21
										22
										23
										24
										25
										26
										27
										28
										29
										30

<table>
<tr><td rowspan="2"></td><td colspan="8" align="center">LOG
Supervised Clinical Practice
Emergency / Prehospital Ultrasound</td></tr>
<tr></tr>
<tr><td></td><td colspan="2" align="center">eFAST</td><td colspan="2" align="center">AAA
(Aorta)</td><td colspan="2" align="center">Vascular Access</td><td colspan="2" align="center">Echo in Life Support</td></tr>
<tr><td>1</td><td>Date</td><td>Sign</td><td>Date</td><td>Sign</td><td>Date</td><td>Sign</td><td>Date</td><td>Sign</td></tr>
<tr><td>2</td><td></td><td></td><td></td><td></td><td></td><td></td><td></td><td></td></tr>
<tr><td>3</td><td></td><td></td><td></td><td></td><td></td><td></td><td></td><td></td></tr>
<tr><td>4</td><td></td><td></td><td></td><td></td><td></td><td></td><td></td><td></td></tr>
<tr><td>5</td><td></td><td></td><td></td><td></td><td></td><td></td><td></td><td></td></tr>
<tr><td>6</td><td></td><td></td><td></td><td></td><td></td><td></td><td></td><td></td></tr>
<tr><td>7</td><td></td><td></td><td></td><td></td><td></td><td></td><td></td><td></td></tr>
<tr><td>8</td><td></td><td></td><td></td><td></td><td></td><td></td><td></td><td></td></tr>
<tr><td>9</td><td></td><td></td><td></td><td></td><td></td><td></td><td></td><td></td></tr>
<tr><td>10</td><td></td><td></td><td></td><td></td><td></td><td></td><td></td><td></td></tr>
<tr><td>11</td><td></td><td></td><td></td><td></td><td></td><td></td><td></td><td></td></tr>
<tr><td>12</td><td></td><td></td><td></td><td></td><td></td><td></td><td></td><td></td></tr>
<tr><td>13</td><td></td><td></td><td></td><td></td><td></td><td></td><td></td><td></td></tr>
<tr><td>14</td><td></td><td></td><td></td><td></td><td></td><td></td><td></td><td></td></tr>
<tr><td>15</td><td></td><td></td><td></td><td></td><td></td><td></td><td></td><td></td></tr>
<tr><td>16</td><td></td><td></td><td></td><td></td><td></td><td></td><td></td><td></td></tr>
<tr><td>17</td><td></td><td></td><td></td><td></td><td></td><td></td><td></td><td></td></tr>
<tr><td>18</td><td></td><td></td><td></td><td></td><td></td><td></td><td></td><td></td></tr>
<tr><td>19</td><td></td><td></td><td></td><td></td><td></td><td></td><td></td><td></td></tr>
<tr><td>20</td><td></td><td></td><td></td><td></td><td></td><td></td><td></td><td></td></tr>
<tr><td>21</td><td></td><td></td><td></td><td></td><td></td><td></td><td></td><td></td></tr>
<tr><td>22</td><td></td><td></td><td></td><td></td><td></td><td></td><td></td><td></td></tr>
<tr><td>23</td><td></td><td></td><td></td><td></td><td></td><td></td><td></td><td></td></tr>
<tr><td>24</td><td></td><td></td><td></td><td></td><td></td><td></td><td></td><td></td></tr>
<tr><td>25</td><td></td><td></td><td></td><td></td><td></td><td></td><td></td><td></td></tr>
<tr><td>26</td><td></td><td></td><td></td><td></td><td></td><td></td><td></td><td></td></tr>
<tr><td>27</td><td></td><td></td><td></td><td></td><td></td><td></td><td></td><td></td></tr>
<tr><td>28</td><td></td><td></td><td></td><td></td><td></td><td></td><td></td><td></td></tr>
<tr><td>29</td><td></td><td></td><td></td><td></td><td></td><td></td><td></td><td></td></tr>
<tr><td>30</td><td></td><td></td><td></td><td></td><td></td><td></td><td></td><td></td></tr>
</table>

LOG
Supervised Clinical Practice
Emergency / Prehospital Ultrasound

IVC (Vena Cava) Measurement		ICP ONSD (Optic Nerve)		Nerve Block		RUSH		Rapid DVT		
Date	Sign	Date	Sign	Date	Sign	Date	Sign	Date	Sign	1
										2
										3
										4
										5
										6
										7
										8
										9
										10
										11
										12
										13
										14
										15
										16
										17
										18
										19
										20
										21
										22
										23
										24
										25
										26
										27
										28
										29
										30

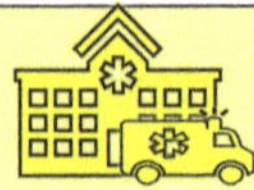

LOG
Independent Clinical Practice
Emergency / Prehospital Ultrasound

	eFAST		AAA (Aorta)		Vascular Access		Echo in Life Support	
1	*Date*	*Sign*	*Date*	*Sign*	*Date*	*Sign*	*Date*	*Sign*
2								
3								
4								
5								
6								
7								
8								
9								
10								
11								
12								
13								
14								
15								
16								
17								
18								
19								
20								
21								
22								
23								
24								
25								
26								
27								
28								
29								
30								

LOG
Independent Clinical Practice
Emergency / Prehospital Ultrasound

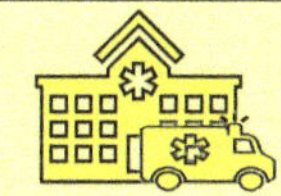

IVC (Vena Cava) Measurement		ICP ONSD (Optic Nerve)		Nerve Block		RUSH		Rapid DVT		
Date	Sign	Date	Sign	Date	Sign	Date	Sign	Date	Sign	1
										2
										3
										4
										5
										6
										7
										8
										9
										10
										11
										12
										13
										14
										15
										16
										17
										18
										19
										20
										21
										22
										23
										24
										25
										26
										27
										28
										29
										30

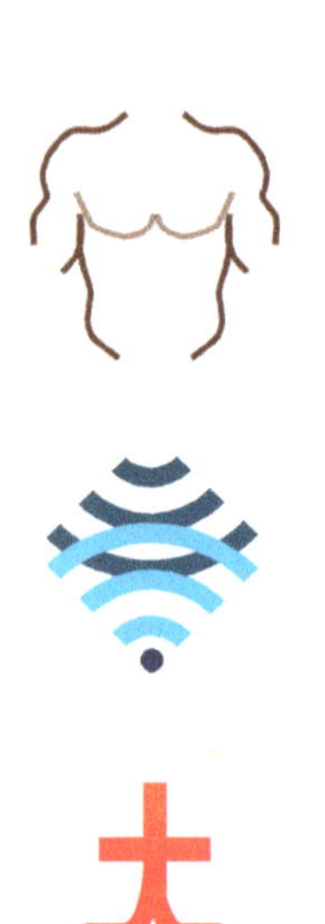
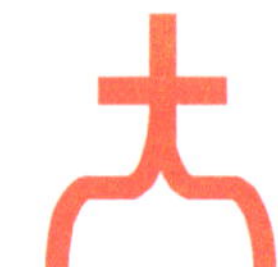
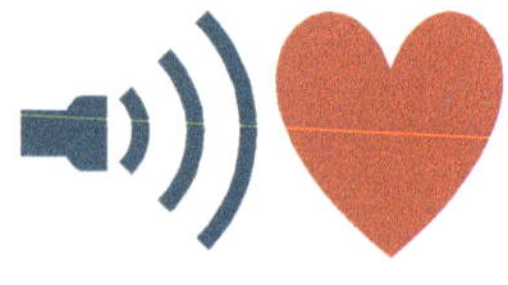
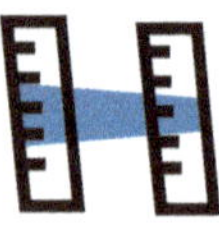
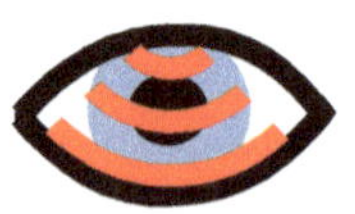
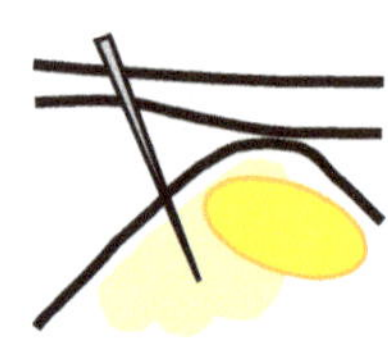
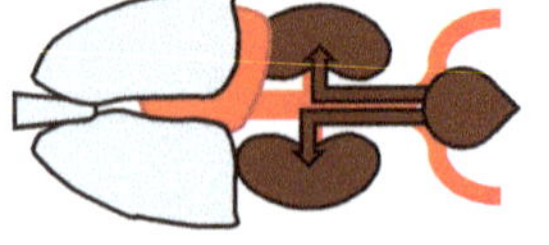
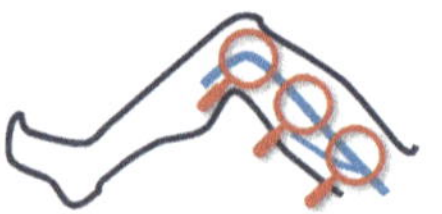

QUICK GUIDES

Extended Focused Assessment with
Sonography in Trauma (eFAST)

Aorta (AAA)

Vascular Access

Echo in Life Support

Inferior Vena Cava (IVC)

Optic Nerve Sheath Diameter (ONSD)

Nerve Block

Rapid Ultrasound for Shock & Hypotension (RUSH)

Rapid DVT Protocol

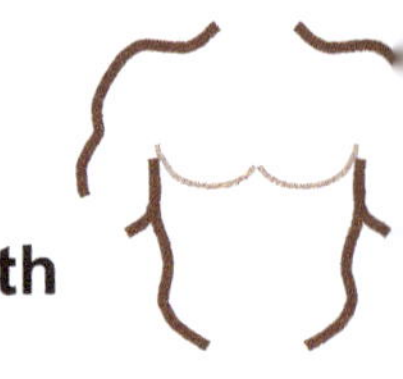

Quick Guide:
Extended Focused Assessment with Sonography in Trauma (eFAST)

	Probe Type	Orientation	Location	Key findings
Lung Right	Linear	Perpendicular to ribs. Orientation marker pointing cephalad.	2nd or 3rd intercostal space to the right of the sternum (can scan anywhere on thorax)	**Normal:** Pleural sliding A- & B-Lines Seashore sign (M-Mode). **Abnormal:** No pleural sliding. No A- & B-Lines Barcode sign (M-Mode).
Lung Left			2nd or 3rd intercostal space to the left of the sternum (can scan anywhere on thorax)	
Cardiac	Curvilinear or phased array	Orientation marker pointing to patient's left. Subcostal view. *See pg 20.*	Transverse in subcostal region to right of sternum, held almost flat to skin & directed towards left shoulder.	**Normal:** Lack of hypoechoic (black) fluid around heart. **Abnormal:** Hypoechoic (black) fluid surrounding heart: *beware epicardial fat pad around RV.*
RUQ		Longitudinal (sagittal) with orientation marker cephalad.	8th-11th intercostal space posterior to midaxillary line.	**Normal:** Hepato-Renal interface. **Abnormal:** Hypoechoic (black) fluid at this interface.
LUQ		Longitudinal (sagittal) with orientation marker cephalad.	6th-10th intercostal space posterior to midaxillary line.	**Normal:** Spleno-Renal interface. **Abnormal:** Hypoechoic (black) fluid at this interface.
Bladder		Transverse with orientation marker to patient's right; then longitudinal (sagittal) with orientation marker cephalad.	Superior to symphysis pubis.	**Normal:** Anterior bladder with hypoechoic (black) fluid within. Rectovesicular or uterovesicular interface. **Abnormal:** Hypoechoic (black) fluid at the interface behind the bladder.

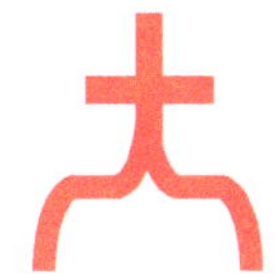

Quick Guide:
Aorta (AAA)

When undertaking aortic scanning as part of a formal screening process, follow local protocols.

A curvilinear probe is usually used. Start your Aortic imaging with a survey scan, scanning the length of the abdominal aorta in longitudinal & transverse orientations.

Measurements are taken at right angles from the anterior to the posterior outer vessel walls. A normal diameter is <3cm.

Be aware of the Cylinder Effect: viewing the aorta off-centre will produce a smaller false diameter. Shown below; diameter A is the true diameter, while diameter B will show a much smaller false diameter.

Longitudinal and transverse measurements should be taken. A fair degree of compression will be required to move bowel gas out of the way, resulting in better image acquisition. Ensure images and measurements are obtained for the widest part of the aorta that you visualise.

Proximal, Mid and Distal measurements should be obtained:

Proximal-Aorta:
Apply the probe in the epigastrium inferior to the xiphoid process, using the left lobe of the liver as an acoustic window.

Mid-Aorta:
Obtained just distal to the branching of the superior mesenteric artery.

Distal-Aorta:
Obtained just prior to the aortic bifurcation.

Common-Iliac Vessels:
These can be included.
They should measure <1.5cm (women) & <1.8cm (men)

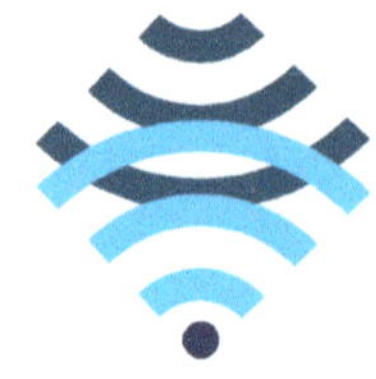

Quick Guide:
Vascular Access

Ultrasound can be a powerful tool for gaining vascular access.

A high frequency linear probe with sterile cover should be utilised, as this will best visualise superficial structures.

When considering make and model of ultrasound, consider purchasing one which provides multi-planar visualisation. This will allow you to view the vessel in the longitudinal and transverse views simultaneously while gaining vascular access.

Once a suitable vessel has been identified, it is good practice to ensure no other neurovascular structures or key elements of the locomotor system (i.e. tendons) are near the intended path of the cannula. It is also prudent to scan some distance along the intended vessel to search for any valves, which can then be avoided.

Remember:
    Veins are usually oval and compressible while arteries are round, less compressible and are pulsatile. Excessive pressure may collapse your venous target.

Activating colour doppler may aid in differentiating the two.
    When used, Blue colour indicates movement away from the probe, and Red colour indicated movement towards the probe.

B.A.R.T.
Blue Away : Red Towards

Contraindications:

- Infection at point of needle insertion
- Distorted anatomy

Complications:

- Bleeding or bruising
- Damage to underlying structures
- Infection
- Air embolism
- Failure

Quick Guide: Echo in Life Support

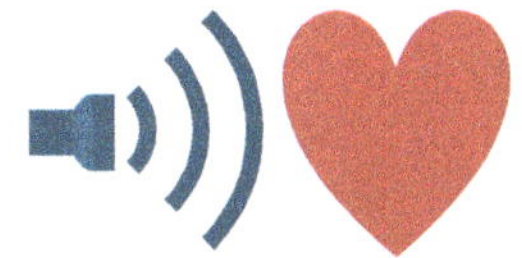

Keep decision-making simple when using point of care ultrasound during cardiac arrest and minimise interruptions to chest compressions.

Subcostal / Subxiphoid view **plus one other view:**

- Apical four chamber (A4C) view
- Parasternal Short Axis (PSAX) view
- Parasternal Long Axis (PLAX) view

See page 20 for larger views

Record a short video during a pause in CPR, then step away to analyse it.

Diagnostic checklist:

1. Is there co-ordinated cardiac activity?
2. Is there a pericardial effusion or tamponade?
3. What is the relative right and left ventricular chamber size?
4. What is overall LV function like?

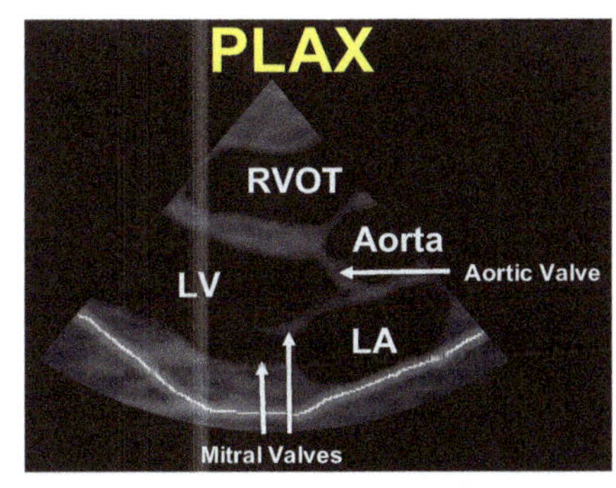

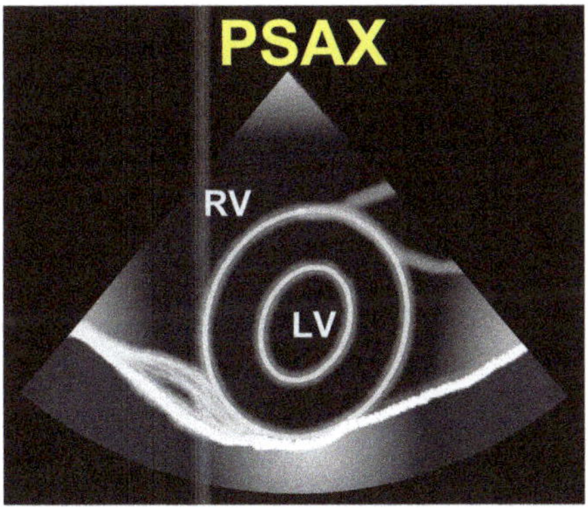

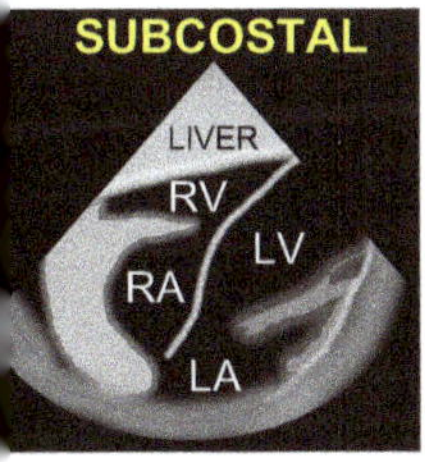

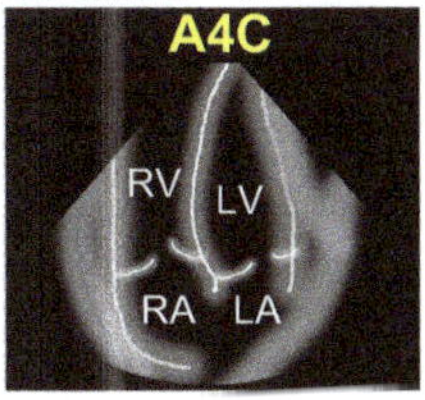

Quick Guide:
Inferior Vena Cava (IVC)

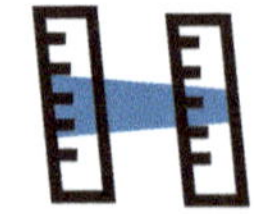

Probe Type	Orientation	Location	Key findings
Curvilinear or phased array	Indicator cephalad. Sagittal view.	Below the costal margin just to the right of the midline	**Identify:** The junction of the IVC and Right Atrium and the middle hepatic vein (to ensure visualisation of the IVC). Measure diameter at a fixed distance from the IVC : atrial junction (~2cm distal).
		Identify the liver, use this as an acoustic window to view the IVC	

Longitudinal ultrasound assessment of the inferior vena cava seeks to identify whether a patient is intravascularly fluid deplete. However, there is no universal agreement on how this assessment should be performed.

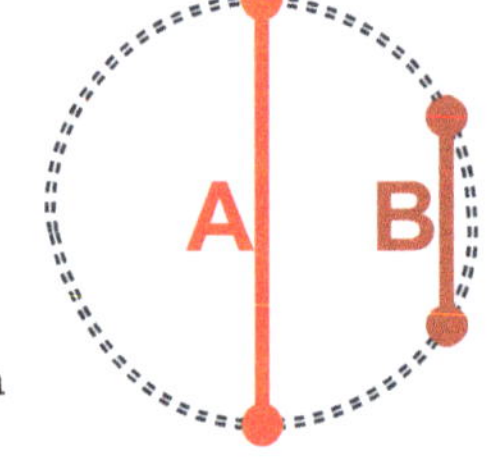

Be aware of the Cylinder Effect. Viewing the IVC off-centre will produce a false diameter, which will be much smaller than the true diameter. Shown here, diameter A is the true diameter, while diameter B will should a much smaller false diameter.

In those who are intravascularly deplete the IVC will appear flat or will collapse. In those with fluid overload or downstream occlusion (e.g. cardiac tamponade or massive PE) the IVC will appear dilated. In conscious patients, collapsibility can be assessed using the "sniff test"; ask your patient to sniff to induce collapsibility.

Inferior vena cava collapsibility index (IVCCI)

Max	Min	Calculation	Collapsibility
_____cm	_____cm	[(Max-Min) / Max] x 100 =	_______%

IVCCI in a Clinical Context?

Ventilation Type	
Spontaneous	**IPPV**
>75% = Depleted	>20% = Depleted
<10-25% = Replete **or** Overload	<10% = Replete **or** Overload

The percentages quoted here are <u>not</u> universally agreed, the art and science of IVC measurement lacks consistent data on which to build a diagnostic consensus.

Quick Guide:
Optic Nerve Sheath Diameter (ONSD)

- A high frequency linear probe (5-18 MHz) is selected.
    - Ensure the chosen probe is safe for ocular ultrasound (*e.g. Butterfly IQ / IQ+ / IQ3*).
- Contraindications:
    - open globe injury, visible conjunctival/scleral defect, severe chemosis, 360-degree conjunctival haemorrhage, hypotony, large hyphema.
- The patient is directed to keep their eyes closed, and sterile ultrasound gel is placed on their closed eyelid. *Alternatively, clingfilm can be applied over the patient's closed eye; non-sterile gel can then be used.*
- The probe is then applied to the gel while the operator anchors their hand to the patient's forehead, orbit or nasal bone to avoid pressure being applied to the patient's globe.
- The probe is manipulated to gain the best view of the optic nerve sheath using transverse or sagittal views. *Ensure the anterior chamber, lens and posterior chamber are in view to avoid gaining an oblique view of the optic nerve sheath.*

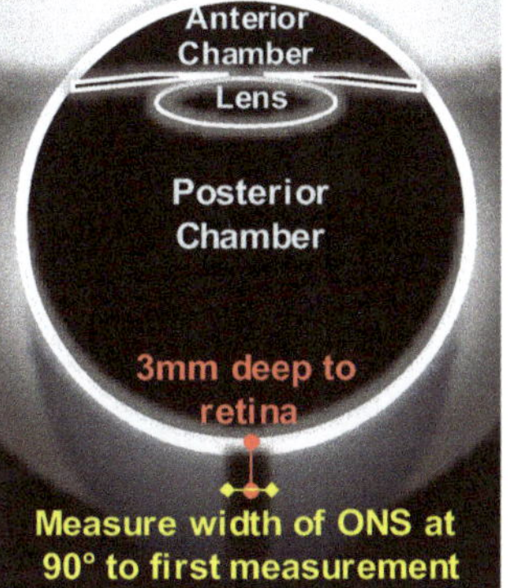

- **Take 2 measurements:**
    1) **Measurement 1** is used to locate how deep to the retina you will measure the diameter of the optic nerve sheath.
        a. Measure 3 mm posterior to the globe.
    2) **Measurement 2** is the measured optic nerve sheath diameter (ONSD).
        a. A normal ONSD is ≤5mm (in adults and children, for infants it is ≤4mm).

- Optic nerve sheath diameter >5mm appears to have diagnostic sensitivity of 95.6% and specificity of 92.3% for raised intracranial pressure (Ohle et al 2015).
- An optic nerve sheath diameter of >5mm appears to correlate well with an intracranial pressure >20 mmHg.
- Elevation of the optic disc of >6mm has a sensitivity of around 82% and a specificity of about 76% for Papilloedema (Teismann et al 2013).

Ohle R, McIsaac SM, Woo MY, Perry JJ. Sonography of the Optic Nerve Sheath Diameter for Detection of Raised Intracranial Pressure Compared to Computed Tomography: A Systematic Review and Meta-analysis. *J Ultrasound Med.* 2015 Jul;34(7):1285-94.

Teismann, N., Lenaghan, P., Nolan, R., Stein, J., & Green, A. (2013). Point-of-care ocular ultrasound to detect optic disc swelling. *Academic Emergency Medicine, 20*(9), 920-925.

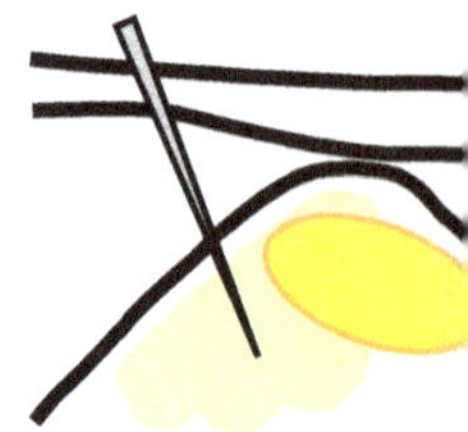

Quick Guide: Ultrasound Guided Nerve Block

Prehospital nerve blocks are gaining popularity. The most commonly used are probably the Fascia Iliaca Compartment Block (FICB) and the Femoral Nerve Block (FNB). Other nerve blocks may be used, and there is increasingly interest in the Serratus Anterior Plane Block (SAPB) for patients with multiple rib fractures.

All ultrasound guided nerve blocks require the same process to ensure safety, and the needle should be fully visualised at all times.

Contraindications:
- Infection at point of needle insertion
- Distorted anatomy
- Allergy to local anaesthetic

Complications:
- Bleeding or bruising
- Damage to underlying structures
- Infection
- Failure
- Local anaesthetic systemic toxicity (LAST)

Prior to Blocking:
- Obtain consent
- Ensure resuscitation equipment to hand
- Calculate local anaesthetic dose (and maximum safe dose)
- Calculate Intralipid dose
- Gain intravascular access
- Apply monitoring (ECG, NiBP, SpO_2)
- Ensure aseptic technique (this may require a sterile probe cover)

STOP BEFORE YOU BLOCK

PREP		STOP		BLOCK
Prepare local anaesthetic		Stop before you block		Perform block
Prepare and label in a tray. Hand tray to Assistant.	→	Proceduralist and Assistant check block site, check with the patient and verbalise this check.	→	Assistant returns tray to the Proceduralist. Perform the block.

Adapted from: https://www.ra-uk.org/

Quick Guide:
Rapid Ultrasound for Shock & Hypotension (RUSH)

		Probe	Orientation	Location	Key findings
Tank	Lung Right / Lung Left	Linear	Perpendicular to ribs. Orientation marker pointing cephalad.	2nd or 3rd intercostal space to the right or left of the sternum (can scan anywhere on thorax)	**Normal:** Pleural sliding A- & B-Lines Seashore sign (M-Mode) **Abnormal:** No pleural sliding No A- & B-Lines Barcode sign (M-Mode)
Pump	Cardiac	Curvilinear or phased array	Orientation marker pointing to patient's left. Subcostal view.	Transverse in subcostal region to right of sternum, held almost flat to skin & directed towards left shoulder.	**Normal:** Lack of hypoechoic (black) fluid around heart **Abnormal:** Hypoechoic (black) fluid surrounding heart: *beware epicardial fat pad around RV*
Tank	RUQ		Longitudinal (sagittal), orientation marker cephalad.	8th-11th intercostal space anterior to the midaxillary line.	**Normal:** Hepato-Renal interface **Abnormal:** Hypoechoic (black) fluid at this interface
Tank	LUQ			6th-10th intercostal space anterior to the midaxillary line.	**Normal:** Spleno-Renal interface **Abnormal:** Hypoechoic (black) fluid at this interface
Tank	Bladder		Transverse, orientation marker to patient's right; & longitudinal (sagittal) with orientation marker cephalad.	Superior to symphysis pubis.	**Normal:** Anterior bladder with hypoechoic (black) fluid within. Rectovesicular or uterovesicular interface **Abnormal:** Hypoechoic (black) fluid at the interface behind the bladder
Pipes	Aorta		A survey scan of the length of the abdominal aorta in longitudinal & transverse orientations.		**Normal:** Aortic diameter <3cm throughout
Pipes	IVC		Indicator cephalad. Sagittal view.	Below the costal margin just to the right of the midline.	Assessment of whether IVC appears: **"Fat"** (Fluid replete/overloaded) or **"Flat"** (deplete)

Quick Guide:
Rapid DVT Protocol

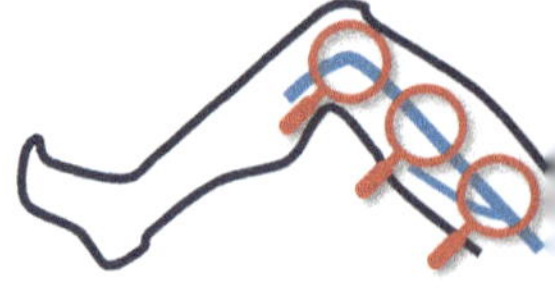

DVT scanning protocols are deployed as a result of high clinical gestalt, Wells score and clinical findings. They are sometimes incorporated as part of the RUSH protocol. There is a <u>rare</u> adverse incident where this ultrasound protocol *may* dislodge a DVT leading to a pulmonary embolus.

Preparation
- Consider elevating the head of the bed by 30° to aid blood pooling in legs.
- Externally rotate the patient's hip and flex the knee "frog leg position".
- Place a pillow under the knee.

We recommend a three-stage examination:

Common Femoral Vein
Compress the Common Femoral Vein (CFV) 2cm above and below the saphenofemoral junction.

Femoral Vein
Compress the Femoral Vein (FV) 2cm above and below of the bifurcation of the common femoral vein into the deep femoral vein and the *superficial* femoral vein.

Popliteal Vein
Compress the Popliteal Vein (PV), located between the two hamstring tendons, down to the trifurcation into the anterior tibial vein, posterior tibial vein, and the peroneal vein. This trifurcation can be targeted and compressed as well.

Use a linear probe with vascular pre-set. Ensure placement is perpendicular to the vein, providing a transverse view. Apply pressure until a visible pulsatile artery is compressed slightly. If the visible vein compresses completely this is reassuring re: a lack of DVT. A thrombus may be visualised within the vein lumen. Colour doppler can be used to identify lack of flow through a vein.

	Fully Compressible	Occlusive Thrombus	Non-Occlusive Thrombus
Common Femoral Vein Right	YES / NO	YES / NO	YES / NO
Common Femoral Vein Left	YES / NO	YES / NO	YES / NO
Femoral Vein Right	YES / NO	YES / NO	YES / NO
Femoral Vein Left	YES / NO	YES / NO	YES / NO
Popliteal Vein Right	YES / NO	YES / NO	YES / NO
Popliteal Vein Left	YES / NO	YES / NO	YES / NO

Cardiac Views Aide Mémoire

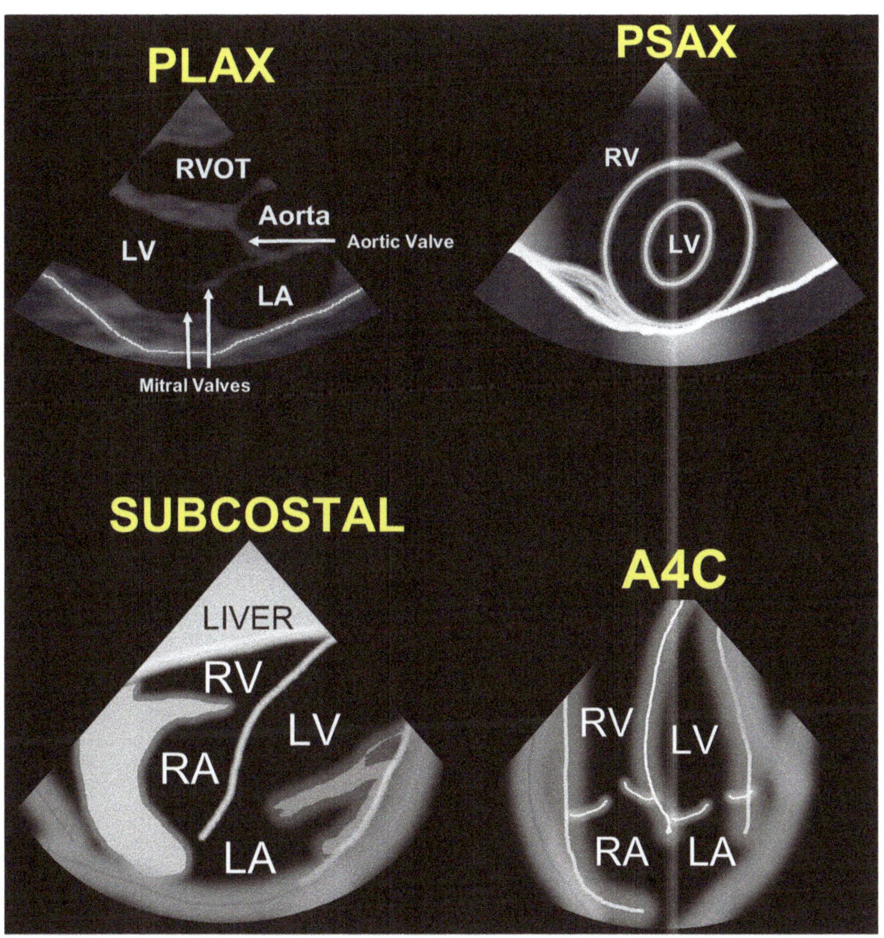

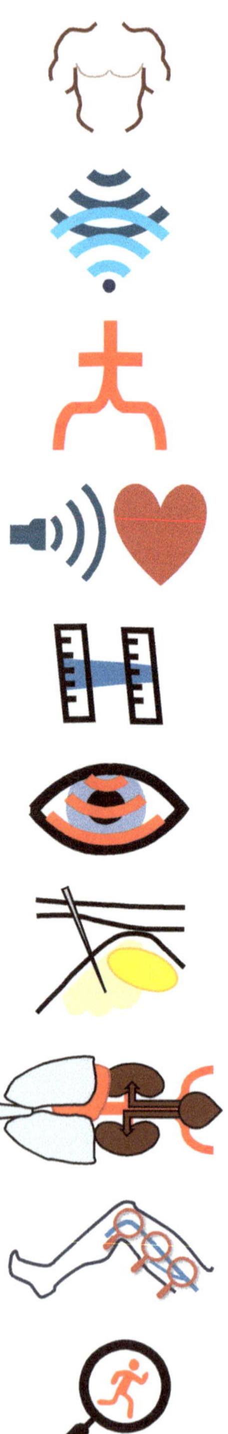

REFLECTIVE CASES
(5 templates for each modality)

Extended Focused Assessment with
Sonography in Trauma (eFAST)

Aorta (AAA)

Vascular Access

Echo In Life Support

Inferior Vena Cava (IVC) Measurement

Optic Nerve Sheath Diameter (ONSD)

Nerve Block

Rapid Ultrasound for Shock & Hypotension (RUSH)

Rapid DVT Protocol

Generic Reflective Template

EFAST
Case Study 1

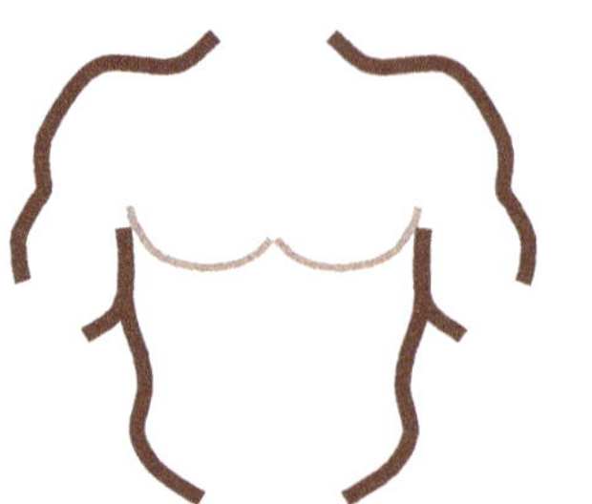

	Anonymised Patient Demographics		
Age:		**Sex:**	
Indication:			

	Image Quality (circle)	**Clinical finding** (circle)
Lung Right	Inadequate → Poor → Good → Excellent	Normal / Abnormal
Lung Left	Inadequate → Poor → Good → Excellent	Normal / Abnormal
Cardiac	Inadequate → Poor → Good → Excellent	Normal / Abnormal
LUQ	Inadequate → Poor → Good → Excellent	Normal / Abnormal
RUQ	Inadequate → Poor → Good → Excellent	Normal / Abnormal
Bladder	Inadequate → Poor → Good → Excellent	Normal / Abnormal

Abnormal clinical findings confirmed on subsequent imaging?	Yes / No / N/A

Practitioner Reflection

Provisional Diagnosis/Interpretation:

Supervisor Comments

Supervisor's Diagnosis/Interpretation:

EFAST
Case Study 2

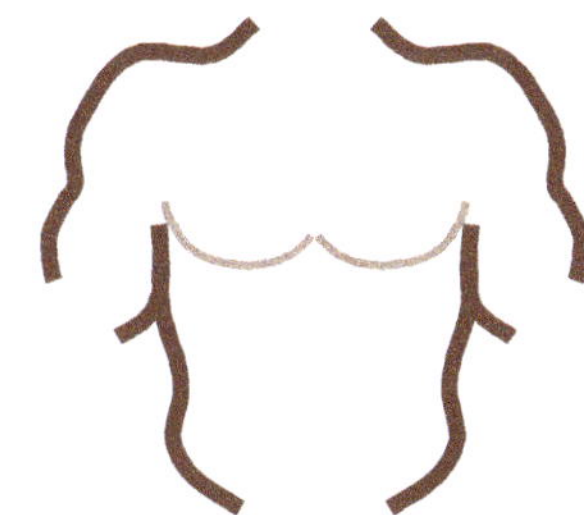

Anonymised Patient Demographics			
Age:		**Sex:**	
Indication:			

	Image Quality (circle)	**Clinical finding** (circle)
Lung Right	Inadequate → Poor → Good → Excellent	Normal / Abnormal
Lung Left	Inadequate → Poor → Good → Excellent	Normal / Abnormal
Cardiac	Inadequate → Poor → Good → Excellent	Normal / Abnormal
LUQ	Inadequate → Poor → Good → Excellent	Normal / Abnormal
RUQ	Inadequate → Poor → Good → Excellent	Normal / Abnormal
Bladder	Inadequate → Poor → Good → Excellent	Normal / Abnormal

Abnormal clinical findings confirmed on subsequent imaging?	Yes / No / N/A

Practitioner Reflection

Provisional Diagnosis/Interpretation:

Supervisor Comments

Supervisor's Diagnosis/Interpretation:

EFAST
Case Study 3

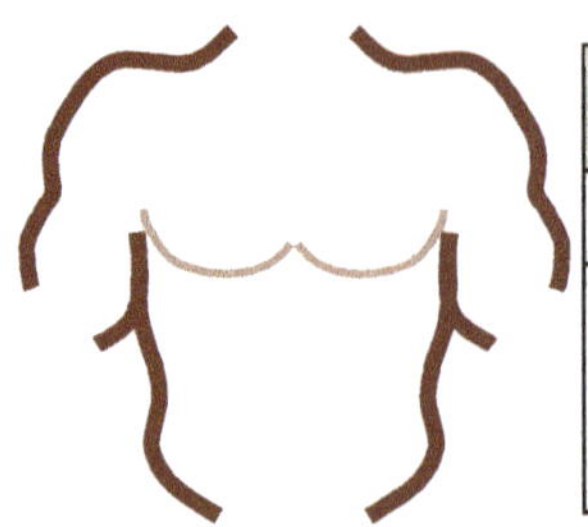

	Anonymised Patient Demographics	
Age:		**Sex:**
Indication:		

	Image Quality (circle)	**Clinical finding** (circle)
Lung Right	Inadequate → Poor → Good → Excellent	Normal / Abnormal
Lung Left	Inadequate → Poor → Good → Excellent	Normal / Abnormal
Cardiac	Inadequate → Poor → Good → Excellent	Normal / Abnormal
LUQ	Inadequate → Poor → Good → Excellent	Normal / Abnormal
RUQ	Inadequate → Poor → Good → Excellent	Normal / Abnormal
Bladder	Inadequate → Poor → Good → Excellent	Normal / Abnormal

Abnormal clinical findings confirmed on subsequent imaging?	Yes / No / N/A

Practitioner Reflection

Provisional Diagnosis/Interpretation:

Supervisor Comments

Supervisor's Diagnosis/Interpretation:

EFAST
Case Study 4

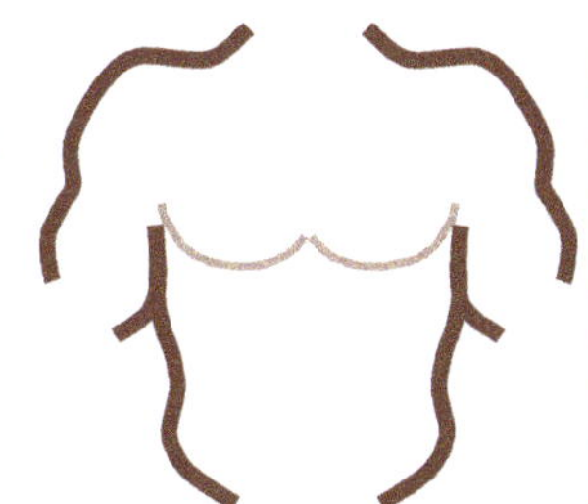

<table>
<tr><td colspan="2">Anonymised Patient Demographics</td></tr>
<tr><td>Age:</td><td></td><td>Sex:</td><td></td></tr>
<tr><td colspan="4">Indication:</td></tr>
</table>

	Image Quality (circle)	**Clinical finding** (circle)
Lung Right	Inadequate → Poor → Good → Excellent	Normal / Abnormal
Lung Left	Inadequate → Poor → Good → Excellent	Normal / Abnormal
Cardiac	Inadequate → Poor → Good → Excellent	Normal / Abnormal
LUQ	Inadequate → Poor → Good → Excellent	Normal / Abnormal
RUQ	Inadequate → Poor → Good → Excellent	Normal / Abnormal
Bladder	Inadequate → Poor → Good → Excellent	Normal / Abnormal

Abnormal clinical findings confirmed on subsequent imaging?	Yes / No / N/A

Practitioner Reflection

Provisional Diagnosis/Interpretation:

Supervisor Comments

Supervisor's Diagnosis/Interpretation:

EFAST
Case Study 5

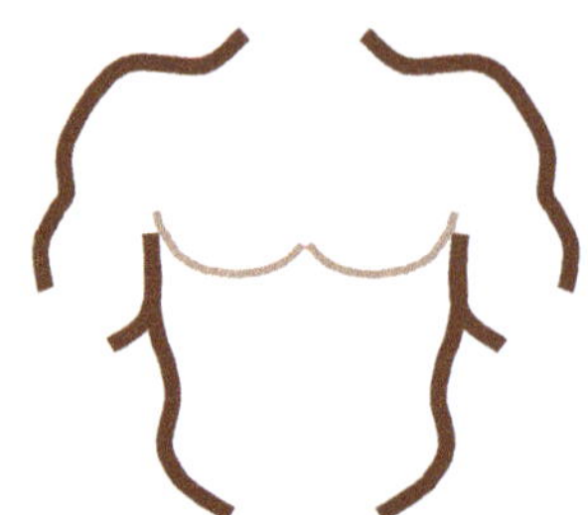

	Anonymised Patient Demographics	
Age:		**Sex:**	
Indication:			

	Image Quality (circle)	**Clinical finding** (circle)
Lung Right	Inadequate → Poor → Good → Excellent	Normal / Abnormal
Lung Left	Inadequate → Poor → Good → Excellent	Normal / Abnormal
Cardiac	Inadequate → Poor → Good → Excellent	Normal / Abnormal
LUQ	Inadequate → Poor → Good → Excellent	Normal / Abnormal
RUQ	Inadequate → Poor → Good → Excellent	Normal / Abnormal
Bladder	Inadequate → Poor → Good → Excellent	Normal / Abnormal

Abnormal clinical findings confirmed on subsequent imaging?	Yes / No / N/A

Practitioner Reflection

Provisional Diagnosis/Interpretation:

Supervisor Comments

Supervisor's Diagnosis/Interpretation:

AORTA (AAA)
Case Study 1

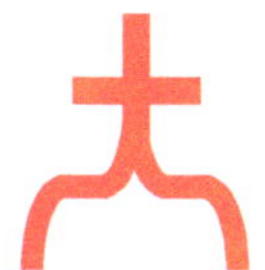

Anonymised Patient Demographics			
Age:		**Sex:**	
Indication:			

Abdominal Aorta	Image Quality (circle)	Clinical finding (circle)
Proximal (*Transverse*)	Inadequate → Adequate	<3cm / 3 – 4.4cm 4.5 – 5.4cm / ≥5.5cm
Proximal (*Longitudinal*)	Inadequate → Adequate	Normal / Abnormal
Mid (*Transverse*)	Inadequate → Adequate	<3cm / 3 – 4.4cm 4.5 – 5.4cm / ≥5.5cm
Mid (*Longitudinal*)	Inadequate → Adequate	Normal / Abnormal
Distal (*Transverse*)	Inadequate → Adequate	<3cm / 3 – 4.4cm 4.5 – 5.4cm / ≥5.5cm
Distal (*Longitudinal*)	Inadequate → Adequate	Normal / Abnormal

Abnormal clinical findings confirmed on subsequent imaging?	Yes / No / N/A

Practitioner Reflection
Provisional Diagnosis/Interpretation:

Supervisor Comments
Supervisor's Diagnosis/Interpretation:

AORTA (AAA)
Case Study 2

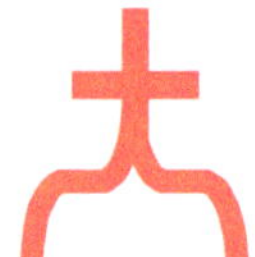

Anonymised Patient Demographics		
Age:		**Sex:**
Indication:		

Abdominal Aorta	Image Quality (circle)	Clinical finding (circle)
Proximal (*Transverse*)	Inadequate → Adequate	<3cm / 3 – 4.4cm 4.5 – 5.4cm / ≥5.5cm
Proximal (*Longitudinal*)	Inadequate → Adequate	Normal / Abnormal
Mid (*Transverse*)	Inadequate → Adequate	<3cm / 3 – 4.4cm 4.5 – 5.4cm / ≥5.5cm
Mid (*Longitudinal*)	Inadequate → Adequate	Normal / Abnormal
Distal (*Transverse*)	Inadequate → Adequate	<3cm / 3 – 4.4cm 4.5 – 5.4cm / ≥5.5cm
Distal (*Longitudinal*)	Inadequate → Adequate	Normal / Abnormal

Abnormal clinical findings confirmed on subsequent imaging?	Yes / No / N/A

Practitioner Reflection

Provisional Diagnosis/Interpretation:

Supervisor Comments

Supervisor's Diagnosis/Interpretation:

AORTA (AAA)
Case Study 3

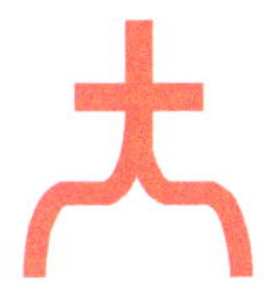

Anonymised Patient Demographics			
Age:		**Sex:**	
Indication:			

Abdominal Aorta	Image Quality (circle)	Clinical finding (circle)
Proximal (*Transverse*)	Inadequate → Adequate	<3cm / 3 – 4.4cm 4.5 – 5.4cm / ≥5.5cm
Proximal (*Longitudinal*)	Inadequate → Adequate	Normal / Abnormal
Mid (*Transverse*)	Inadequate → Adequate	<3cm / 3 – 4.4cm 4.5 – 5.4cm / ≥5.5cm
Mid (*Longitudinal*)	Inadequate → Adequate	Normal / Abnormal
Distal (*Transverse*)	Inadequate → Adequate	<3cm / 3 – 4.4cm 4.5 – 5.4cm / ≥5.5cm
Distal (*Longitudinal*)	Inadequate → Adequate	Normal / Abnormal

Abnormal clinical findings confirmed on subsequent imaging?	Yes / No / N/A

Practitioner Reflection

Provisional Diagnosis/Interpretation:

Supervisor Comments

Supervisor's Diagnosis/Interpretation:

AORTA (AAA)
Case Study 4

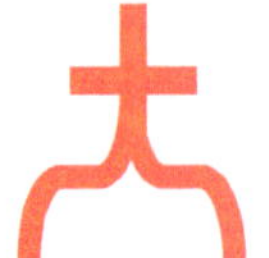

Anonymised Patient Demographics			
Age:		**Sex:**	
Indication:			

Abdominal Aorta	Image Quality (circle)	Clinical finding (circle)
Proximal (*Transverse*)	Inadequate → Adequate	<3cm / 3 – 4.4cm 4.5 – 5.4cm / ≥5.5cm
Proximal (*Longitudinal*)	Inadequate → Adequate	Normal / Abnormal
Mid (*Transverse*)	Inadequate → Adequate	<3cm / 3 – 4.4cm 4.5 – 5.4cm / ≥5.5cm
Mid (*Longitudinal*)	Inadequate → Adequate	Normal / Abnormal
Distal (*Transverse*)	Inadequate → Adequate	<3cm / 3 – 4.4cm 4.5 – 5.4cm / ≥5.5cm
Distal (*Longitudinal*)	Inadequate → Adequate	Normal / Abnormal

Abnormal clinical findings confirmed on subsequent imaging?	Yes / No / N/A

Practitioner Reflection

Provisional Diagnosis/Interpretation:

Supervisor Comments

Supervisor's Diagnosis/Interpretation:

AORTA (AAA)
Case Study 5

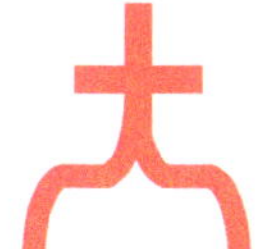

Anonymised Patient Demographics			
Age:		**Sex:**	
Indication:			

Abdominal Aorta	**Image Quality** (circle)	**Clinical finding** (circle)
Proximal (*Transverse*)	Inadequate → Adequate	<3cm / 3 – 4.4cm 4.5 – 5.4cm / ≥5.5cm
Proximal (*Longitudinal*)	Inadequate → Adequate	Normal / Abnormal
Mid (*Transverse*)	Inadequate → Adequate	<3cm / 3 – 4.4cm 4.5 – 5.4cm / ≥5.5cm
Mid (*Longitudinal*)	Inadequate → Adequate	Normal / Abnormal
Distal (*Transverse*)	Inadequate → Adequate	<3cm / 3 – 4.4cm 4.5 – 5.4cm / ≥5.5cm
Distal (*Longitudinal*)	Inadequate → Adequate	Normal / Abnormal

Abnormal clinical findings confirmed on subsequent imaging?	Yes / No / N/A

Practitioner Reflection

Provisional Diagnosis/Interpretation:

Supervisor Comments

Supervisor's Diagnosis/Interpretation:

Vascular Access
Case Study 1

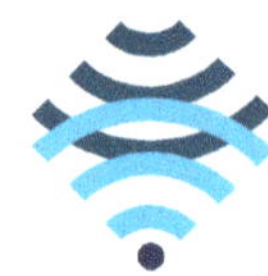

<table>
<tr><td colspan="4">Anonymised Patient Demographics</td></tr>
<tr><td>Age:</td><td></td><td>Sex:</td><td></td></tr>
<tr><td colspan="4">Indication:</td></tr>
</table>

View	Image Quality (circle)
Transverse / Short	Inadequate → Poor → Good → Excellent
Longitudinal / Long	Inadequate → Poor → Good → Excellent
Needle Visualisation	Inadequate → Poor → Good → Excellent

Location	Anatomical Location	Setting	Type	Axis Used for Venepuncture
Peripheral ☐ Central ☐	________	In-Hospital ☐ Pre-Hospital ☐	Sterile ☐ Emergent ☐	Short ☐ Long ☐ Biplane ☐

Vascular access successful?	Yes / No

Practitioner Reflection

Provisional Interpretation:

Supervisor Comments

Supervisor's Interpretation:

Vascular Access
Case Study 2

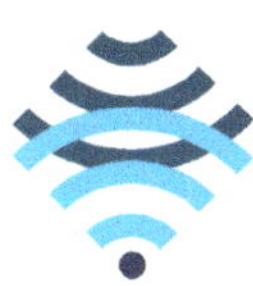

Anonymised Patient Demographics			
Age:		**Sex:**	
Indication:			

View	Image Quality (circle)
Transverse / Short	Inadequate → Poor → Good → Excellent
Longitudinal / Long	Inadequate → Poor → Good → Excellent
Needle Visualisation	Inadequate → Poor → Good → Excellent

Location	Anatomical Location	Setting	Type	Axis Used for Venepuncture
Peripheral ☐ Central ☐	__________	In-Hospital ☐ Pre-Hospital ☐	Sterile ☐ Emergent ☐	Short ☐ Long ☐ Biplane ☐

Vascular access successful?	Yes / No

Practitioner Reflection

Provisional Interpretation:

Supervisor Comments

Supervisor's Interpretation:

Vascular Access
Case Study 3

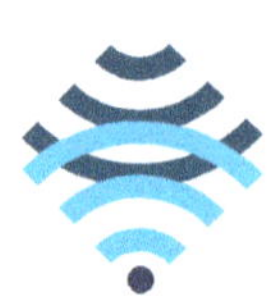

Anonymised Patient Demographics			
Age:		**Sex:**	
Indication:			

View	Image Quality (circle)
Transverse / Short	Inadequate → Poor → Good → Excellent
Longitudinal / Long	Inadequate → Poor → Good → Excellent
Needle Visualisation	Inadequate → Poor → Good → Excellent

Location	Anatomical Location	Setting	Type	Axis Used for Venepuncture
Peripheral ☐ Central ☐	________	In-Hospital ☐ Pre-Hospital ☐	Sterile ☐ Emergent ☐	Short ☐ Long ☐ Biplane ☐

Vascular access successful?	Yes / No

Practitioner Reflection

Provisional Interpretation:

Supervisor Comments

Supervisor's Interpretation:

Vascular Access
Case Study 4

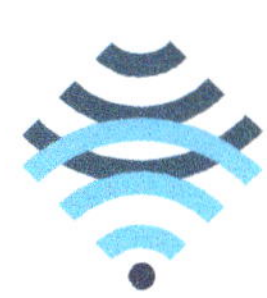

Anonymised Patient Demographics		
Age:		**Sex:**
Indication:		

View	Image Quality (circle)
Transverse / Short	Inadequate → Poor → Good → Excellent
Longitudinal / Long	Inadequate → Poor → Good → Excellent
Needle Visualisation	Inadequate → Poor → Good → Excellent

Location	Anatomical Location	Setting	Type	Axis Used for Venepuncture
Peripheral ☐ Central ☐	______	In-Hospital ☐ Pre-Hospital ☐	Sterile ☐ Emergent ☐	Short ☐ Long ☐ Biplane ☐

Vascular access successful?	Yes / No

Practitioner Reflection

Provisional Interpretation:

Supervisor Comments

Supervisor's Interpretation:

Vascular Access
Case Study 5

Anonymised Patient Demographics			
Age:		**Sex:**	
Indication:			

View	Image Quality (circle)
Transverse / Short	Inadequate → Poor → Good → Excellent
Longitudinal / Long	Inadequate → Poor → Good → Excellent
Needle Visualisation	Inadequate → Poor → Good → Excellent

Location	Anatomical Location	Setting	Type	Axis Used for Venepuncture
Peripheral ☐ Central ☐	__________	In-Hospital ☐ Pre-Hospital ☐	Sterile ☐ Emergent ☐	Short ☐ Long ☐ Biplane ☐

Vascular access successful?	Yes / No

Practitioner Reflection
Provisional Interpretation:

Supervisor Comments
Supervisor's Interpretation:

Echo in Life Support
Case Study 1

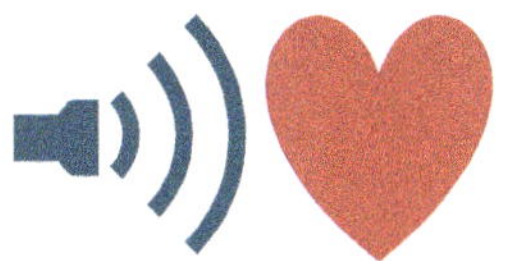

Anonymised Patient Demographics			
Age:		**Sex:**	
Presumed aetiology of arrest: Medical ☐ Traumatic ☐			

Views Obtained	Image Quality (circle)	View Obtained	Image Quality (circle)
PSAX ☐	Inadequate → Adequate	**Apical** ☐	Inadequate → Adequate
PLAX ☐	Inadequate → Adequate	**Subxiphoid** ☐	Inadequate → Adequate

IVC assessment undertaken?	Yes / No

Practitioner Reflection	Supervisor Comments

Echo in Life Support
Case Study 2

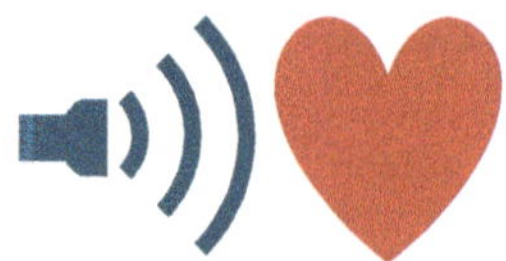

Anonymised Patient Demographics			
Age:		**Sex:**	
Presumed aetiology of arrest: Medical ☐ Traumatic ☐			

Views Obtained	Image Quality (circle)	View Obtained	Image Quality (circle)
PSAX ☐	Inadequate → Adequate	**Apical** ☐	Inadequate → Adequate
PLAX ☐	Inadequate → Adequate	**Subxiphoid** ☐	Inadequate → Adequate

IVC assessment undertaken?	Yes / No

Practitioner Reflection	Supervisor Comments

Echo in Life Support
Case Study 3

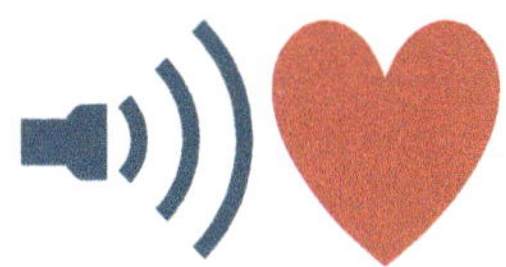

Anonymised Patient Demographics			
Age:		**Sex:**	
Presumed aetiology of arrest: Medical ☐			Traumatic ☐

Views Obtained	Image Quality (circle)	View Obtained	Image Quality (circle)
PSAX ☐	Inadequate → Adequate	**Apical** ☐	Inadequate → Adequate
PLAX ☐	Inadequate → Adequate	**Subxiphoid** ☐	Inadequate → Adequate

IVC assessment undertaken?	Yes / No

Practitioner Reflection	Supervisor Comments

Echo in Life Support
Case Study 4

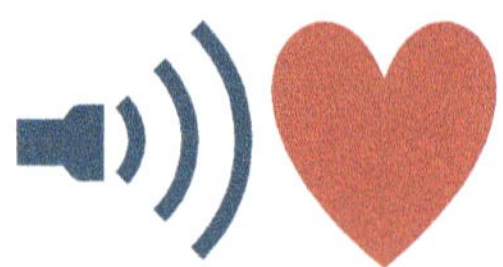

Anonymised Patient Demographics			
Age:		**Sex:**	
Presumed aetiology of arrest: Medical ☐　　　　　Traumatic ☐			

Views Obtained	**Image Quality** (circle)	**View Obtained**	**Image Quality** (circle)
PSAX ☐	Inadequate → Adequate	**Apical** ☐	Inadequate → Adequate
PLAX ☐	Inadequate → Adequate	**Subxiphoid** ☐	Inadequate → Adequate

IVC assessment undertaken?	Yes / No

Practitioner Reflection	**Supervisor Comments**

Echo in Life Support
Case Study 5

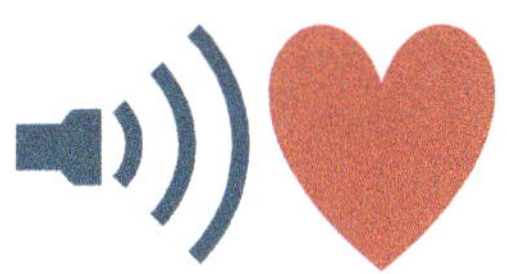

Anonymised Patient Demographics			
Age:		**Sex:**	
Presumed aetiology of arrest: Medical ☐ Traumatic ☐			

Views Obtained	Image Quality (circle)	View Obtained	Image Quality (circle)
PSAX ☐	Inadequate → Adequate	**Apical** ☐	Inadequate → Adequate
PLAX ☐	Inadequate → Adequate	**Subxiphoid** ☐	Inadequate → Adequate

IVC assessment undertaken?	Yes / No

Practitioner Reflection	Supervisor Comments

IVC Measurement
Case Study 1

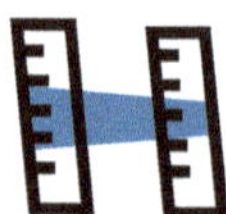

Anonymised Patient Demographics			
Age:		**Sex:**	
Indication:			

IVC	Image Quality (circle)	Clinical finding (circle)
Subxiphoid Longitudinal	Inadequate → Poor → Good → Excellent	Size:____cm

Max	Min	*Calculation*	Collapsibility
____cm	____cm	[(Max-Min) / Max] x 100 =	________%

	Spontaneous	IPPV
Spontaneous ☐ IPPV ☐	>75% = Depleted <25% = Replete or Overload	>20% = Depleted <10% = Replete or Overload

Practitioner Reflection

Provisional Diagnosis/Interpretation:

Supervisor Comments

Supervisor's Diagnosis/Interpretation:

IVC Measurement
Case Study 2

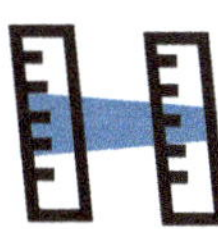

Anonymised Patient Demographics			
Age:		**Sex:**	
Indication:			

IVC	Image Quality (circle)	Clinical finding (circle)
Subxiphoid Longitudinal	Inadequate → Poor → Good → Excellent	Size:____cm

Max	Min	*Calculation*	Collapsibility
____cm	____cm	[(Max-Min) / Max] x 100 =	________%

	Spontaneous	IPPV
Spontaneous ☐ IPPV ☐	>75% = Depleted <25% = Replete or Overload	>20% = Depleted <10% = Replete or Overload

Practitioner Reflection

Provisional Diagnosis/Interpretation:

Supervisor Comments

Supervisor's Diagnosis/Interpretation:

IVC Measurement
Case Study 3

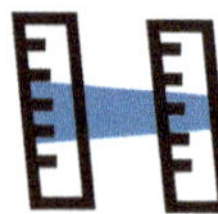

<table>
<tr><td colspan="2">Anonymised Patient Demographics</td></tr>
<tr><td>Age:</td><td>Sex:</td></tr>
<tr><td colspan="2">Indication:</td></tr>
</table>

IVC	**Image Quality** (circle)	**Clinical finding** (circle)
Subxiphoid Longitudinal	Inadequate → Poor → Good → Excellent	Size:____cm

Max	**Min**	*Calculation*	**Collapsibility**
____cm	____cm	[(Max-Min) / Max] x 100 =	_________%

	Spontaneous	**IPPV**
Spontaneous ☐ IPPV ☐	>75% = Depleted <25% = Replete or Overload	>20% = Depleted <10% = Replete or Overload

Practitioner Reflection

Provisional Diagnosis/Interpretation:

Supervisor Comments

Supervisor's Diagnosis/Interpretation:

IVC Measurement
Case Study 4

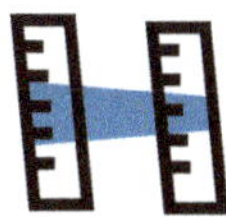

Anonymised Patient Demographics			
Age:		**Sex:**	
Indication:			

IVC	Image Quality (circle)	Clinical finding (circle)
Subxiphoid Longitudinal	Inadequate → Poor → Good → Excellent	Size:____cm

Max	Min	*Calculation*	Collapsibility
____cm	____cm	[(Max-Min) / Max] x 100 =	________%

	Spontaneous	IPPV
Spontaneous ☐ IPPV ☐	>75% = Depleted <25% = Replete or Overload	>20% = Depleted <10% = Replete or Overload

Practitioner Reflection

Provisional Diagnosis/Interpretation:

Supervisor Comments

Supervisor's Diagnosis/Interpretation:

IVC Measurement
Case Study 5

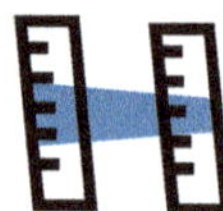

Anonymised Patient Demographics			
Age:		**Sex:**	
Indication:			

IVC	Image Quality (circle)	Clinical finding (circle)
Subxiphoid Longitudinal	Inadequate → Poor → Good → Excellent	Size:_____cm

Max	Min	*Calculation*	Collapsibility
_____cm	_____cm	[(Max-Min) / Max] x 100 =	_________%

	Spontaneous	IPPV
Spontaneous ☐ IPPV ☐	>75% = Depleted <25% = Replete or Overload	>20% = Depleted <10% = Replete or Overload

Practitioner Reflection

Provisional Diagnosis/Interpretation:

Supervisor Comments

Supervisor's Diagnosis/Interpretation:

ICP - ONSD
Case Study 1

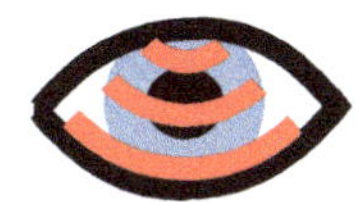

Anonymised Patient Demographics			
Age:		**Sex:**	
Indication:			

	Image Quality (circle)	**ONSD (3mm deep to retina)** (circle)
Right Eye	Inadequate → Adequate	<5mm / >5mm
Left Eye	Inadequate → Adequate	<5mm / >5mm

	Structures Visualised	**Clinical Impression** (circle)
Right Eye	Anterior Chamber ☐ Iris ☐ Lens ☐ Posterior Chamber ☐	Normal / Abnormal
Left Eye	Anterior Chamber ☐ Iris ☐ Lens ☐ Posterior Chamber ☐	Normal / Abnormal

Abnormal clinical findings confirmed on subsequent imaging?	Yes / No / N/A

Practitioner Reflection
Provisional Diagnosis/Interpretation:

Supervisor Comments
Supervisor's Diagnosis/Interpretation:

ICP - ONSD
Case Study 2

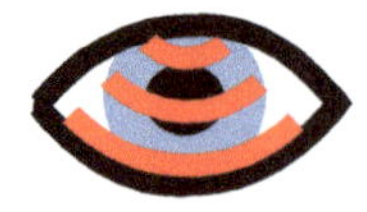

<table>
<tr><td colspan="2">Anonymised Patient Demographics</td></tr>
<tr><td>Age:</td><td>Sex:</td></tr>
<tr><td colspan="2">Indication:</td></tr>
</table>

	Image Quality (circle)	**ONSD (3mm deep to retina)** (circle)
Right Eye	Inadequate → Adequate	<5mm / >5mm
Left Eye	Inadequate → Adequate	<5mm / >5mm

	Structures Visualised	**Clinical Impression** (circle)
Right Eye	Anterior Chamber ☐ Iris ☐ Lens ☐ Posterior Chamber ☐	Normal / Abnormal
Left Eye	Anterior Chamber ☐ Iris ☐ Lens ☐ Posterior Chamber ☐	Normal / Abnormal

Abnormal clinical findings confirmed on subsequent imaging?	Yes / No / N/A

Practitioner Reflection

Provisional Diagnosis/Interpretation:

Supervisor Comments

Supervisor's Diagnosis/Interpretation:

ICP - ONSD
Case Study 3

<table>
<tr><td colspan="2" style="text-align:center">Anonymised Patient Demographics</td></tr>
<tr><td>Age:</td><td>Sex:</td></tr>
<tr><td colspan="2">Indication:</td></tr>
</table>

	Image Quality (circle)	**ONSD (3mm deep to retina)** (circle)
Right Eye	Inadequate → Adequate	<5mm / >5mm
Left Eye	Inadequate → Adequate	<5mm / >5mm

	Structures Visualised	**Clinical Impression** (circle)
Right Eye	Anterior Chamber ☐ Iris ☐　　Lens ☐ Posterior Chamber ☐	Normal / Abnormal
Left Eye	Anterior Chamber ☐ Iris ☐　　Lens ☐ Posterior Chamber ☐	Normal / Abnormal

Abnormal clinical findings confirmed on subsequent imaging?	Yes / No / N/A

Practitioner Reflection

Provisional Diagnosis/Interpretation:

Supervisor Comments

Supervisor's Diagnosis/Interpretation:

ICP - ONSD
Case Study 4

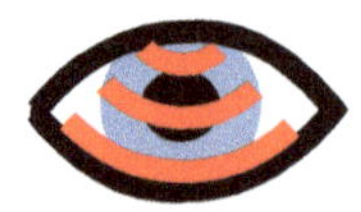

<table>
<tr><th colspan="2" style="background-color:#f0f0e0">Anonymised Patient Demographics</th></tr>
<tr><td>Age:</td><td></td><td>Sex:</td><td></td></tr>
<tr><td colspan="4">Indication:</td></tr>
</table>

	Image Quality (circle)	**ONSD (3mm deep to retina)** (circle)
Right Eye	Inadequate → Adequate	<5mm / >5mm
Left Eye	Inadequate → Adequate	<5mm / >5mm

	Structures Visualised	**Clinical Impression** (circle)
Right Eye	Anterior Chamber ☐ Iris ☐　　　Lens ☐ Posterior Chamber ☐	Normal / Abnormal
Left Eye	Anterior Chamber ☐ Iris ☐　　　Lens ☐ Posterior Chamber ☐	Normal / Abnormal

Abnormal clinical findings confirmed on subsequent imaging?	Yes / No / N/A

Practitioner Reflection

Provisional Diagnosis/Interpretation:

Supervisor Comments

Supervisor's Diagnosis/Interpretation:

ICP - ONSD
Case Study 5

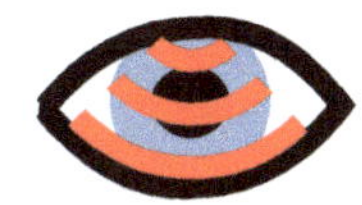

	Anonymised Patient Demographics		
Age:		**Sex:**	
Indication:			

	Image Quality (circle)	**ONSD (3mm deep to retina)** (circle)
Right Eye	Inadequate → Adequate	<5mm / >5mm
Left Eye	Inadequate → Adequate	<5mm / >5mm

	Structures Visualised	**Clinical Impression** (circle)
Right Eye	Anterior Chamber ☐ Iris ☐ Lens ☐ Posterior Chamber ☐	Normal / Abnormal
Left Eye	Anterior Chamber ☐ Iris ☐ Lens ☐ Posterior Chamber ☐	Normal / Abnormal

Abnormal clinical findings confirmed on subsequent imaging?	Yes / No / N/A

Practitioner Reflection
Provisional Diagnosis/Interpretation:

Supervisor Comments
Supervisor's Diagnosis/Interpretation:

Ultrasound Guided Nerve Block

Case Study 1

<table>
<tr><td colspan="2" style="background:#f7f4c0">Anonymised Patient Demographics</td></tr>
<tr><td>Age:</td><td>Sex:</td></tr>
<tr><td colspan="2">Indication:</td></tr>
</table>

Nerve Block:	
Approach:	In-plane / Out-of-plane
Setting:	Prehospital / In-Hospital
Supervision:	Direct / Indirect / Independent

Structure Visualisation	Inadequate → Poor → Good → Excellent
Needle visualisation	Inadequate → Poor → Good → Excellent
Visualisation of needle tip when injecting	Yes / No

Pain Score Pre-Block	0 → 1 → 2 → 3 → 4 → 5 → 6 → 7 → 8 → 9 → 10
Pain Score Post-Block	0 → 1 → 2 → 3 → 4 → 5 → 6 → 7 → 8 → 9 → 10

Patient Weight	Local Anaesthetic Chosen	Max Dose Calculated	Dose Given
____kg			

Additions to Injection:	Steroid:
	Opioid:
	Other:

Calculated dose of Intralipid 20%:	

Initial bolus dose is usually 1.5mL/kg given over 2-3 minutes

Practitioner Reflection	Supervisor Comments

Ultrasound Guided Nerve Block

Case Study 2

<table>
<tr><td colspan="4">Anonymised Patient Demographics</td></tr>
<tr><td>Age:</td><td></td><td>Sex:</td><td></td></tr>
<tr><td colspan="4">Indication:</td></tr>
</table>

Nerve Block:	

Approach:	In-plane / Out-of-plane	Setting:	Prehospital / In-Hospital
Supervision:	Direct / Indirect / Independent		

Structure Visualisation	Inadequate → Poor → Good → Excellent
Needle visualisation	Inadequate → Poor → Good → Excellent
Visualisation of needle tip when injecting	Yes / No

Pain Score Pre-Block	0 → 1 → 2 → 3 → 4 → 5 → 6 → 7 → 8 → 9 → 10
Pain Score Post-Block	0 → 1 → 2 → 3 → 4 → 5 → 6 → 7 → 8 → 9 → 10

Patient Weight	Local Anaesthetic Chosen	Max Dose Calculated	Dose Given
____kg			

Additions to Injection:	Steroid:
	Opioid:
	Other:

Calculated dose of Intralipid 20%:	

Initial bolus dose is usually 1.5mL/kg given over 2-3 minutes

Practitioner Reflection	Supervisor Comments

Ultrasound Guided Nerve Block

Case Study 3

<table>
<tr><td colspan="2">Anonymised Patient Demographics</td></tr>
<tr><td>Age:</td><td>Sex:</td></tr>
<tr><td colspan="2">Indication:</td></tr>
</table>

Nerve Block:	
Approach:	In-plane / Out-of-plane **Setting:** Prehospital / In-Hospital
Supervision:	Direct / Indirect / Independent

Structure Visualisation	Inadequate → Poor → Good → Excellent
Needle visualisation	Inadequate → Poor → Good → Excellent
Visualisation of needle tip when injecting	Yes / No

Pain Score Pre-Block	0 → 1 → 2 → 3 → 4 → 5 → 6 → 7 → 8 → 9 → 10
Pain Score Post-Block	0 → 1 → 2 → 3 → 4 → 5 → 6 → 7 → 8 → 9 → 10

Patient Weight	Local Anaesthetic Chosen	Max Dose Calculated	Dose Given
____kg			

Additions to Injection:	Steroid:
	Opioid:
	Other:

Calculated dose of Intralipid 20%:	

Initial bolus dose is usually 1.5mL/kg given over 2-3 minutes

Practitioner Reflection	Supervisor Comments

Ultrasound Guided Nerve Block

Case Study 4

<table>
<tr><td colspan="4">Anonymised Patient Demographics</td></tr>
<tr><td>Age:</td><td></td><td>Sex:</td><td></td></tr>
<tr><td colspan="4">Indication:</td></tr>
</table>

Nerve Block:	

Approach:	In-plane / Out-of-plane	Setting:	Prehospital / In-Hospital
Supervision:	Direct / Indirect / Independent		

Structure Visualisation	Inadequate → Poor → Good → Excellent
Needle visualisation	Inadequate → Poor → Good → Excellent
Visualisation of needle tip when injecting	Yes / No

Pain Score Pre-Block	0 → 1 → 2 → 3 → 4 → 5 → 6 → 7 → 8 → 9 → 10
Pain Score Post-Block	0 → 1 → 2 → 3 → 4 → 5 → 6 → 7 → 8 → 9 → 10

Patient Weight	Local Anaesthetic Chosen	Max Dose Calculated	Dose Given
_____kg			

Additions to Injection:	Steroid:
	Opioid:
	Other:

Calculated dose of Intralipid 20%:	

Initial bolus dose is usually 1.5mL/kg given over 2-3 minutes

Practitioner Reflection	Supervisor Comments

Ultrasound Guided Nerve Block

Case Study 5

<table>
<tr><td colspan="2">Anonymised Patient Demographics</td></tr>
<tr><td>Age:</td><td>Sex:</td></tr>
<tr><td colspan="2">Indication:</td></tr>
</table>

Nerve Block:	

Approach:	In-plane / Out-of-plane **Setting:** Prehospital / In-Hospital
Supervision:	Direct / Indirect / Independent

Structure Visualisation	Inadequate → Poor → Good → Excellent
Needle visualisation	Inadequate → Poor → Good → Excellent
Visualisation of needle tip when injecting	Yes / No

Pain Score Pre-Block	0 → 1 → 2 → 3 → 4 → 5 → 6 → 7 → 8 → 9 → 10
Pain Score Post-Block	0 → 1 → 2 → 3 → 4 → 5 → 6 → 7 → 8 → 9 → 10

Patient Weight	Local Anaesthetic Chosen	Max Dose Calculated	Dose Given
____kg			

Additions to Injection:	
	Steroid:
	Opioid:
	Other:

Calculated dose of Intralipid 20%:	

Initial bolus dose is usually 1.5mL/kg given over 2-3 minutes

Practitioner Reflection	Supervisor Comments

Rapid Ultrasound for Shock & Hypotension (RUSH)

Case Study 1

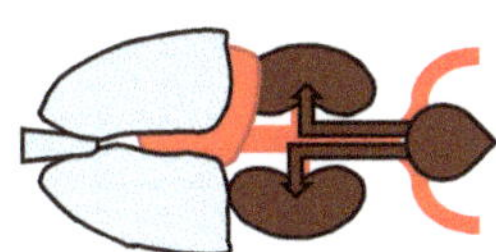

Anonymised Patient Demographics			
Age:		**Sex:**	
Indication:			

	Views	**Image Quality**	**Clinical finding**
Pump	**Cardiac PLAX**	Inadequate → Poor → Good → Excellent	Normal / Abnormal
	Cardiac A4C	Inadequate → Poor → Good → Excellent	Normal / Abnormal
Tank	**Lung Right**	Inadequate → Poor → Good → Excellent	Normal / Abnormal
	Lung Left	Inadequate → Poor → Good → Excellent	Normal / Abnormal
	RUQ	Inadequate → Poor → Good → Excellent	Normal / Abnormal
	LUQ	Inadequate → Poor → Good → Excellent	Normal / Abnormal
	Pelvic	Inadequate → Poor → Good → Excellent	Normal / Abnormal
Pipes	**IVC**	Inadequate → Poor → Good → Excellent	Normal / Abnormal
	Aorta	Inadequate → Poor → Good → Excellent	Normal / Abnormal

Abnormal clinical findings confirmed on subsequent imaging?	Yes / No / N/A

Practitioner Reflection

Provisional Diagnosis/Interpretation:

Supervisor Comments

Supervisor's Diagnosis/Interpretation:

Rapid Ultrasound for Shock & Hypotension (RUSH)

Case Study 2

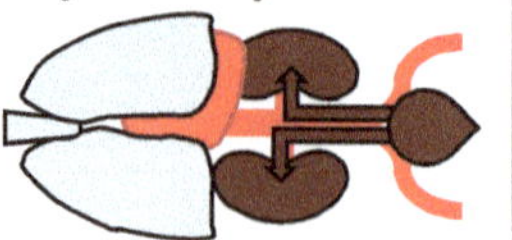

<table>
<tr><td colspan="2">Anonymised Patient Demographics</td></tr>
<tr><td>Age:</td><td>Sex:</td></tr>
<tr><td colspan="2">Indication:</td></tr>
</table>

	Views	Image Quality	Clinical finding
Pump	**Cardiac PLAX**	Inadequate → Poor → Good → Excellent	Normal / Abnormal
	Cardiac A4C	Inadequate → Poor → Good → Excellent	Normal / Abnormal
Tank	**Lung Right**	Inadequate → Poor → Good → Excellent	Normal / Abnormal
	Lung Left	Inadequate → Poor → Good → Excellent	Normal / Abnormal
	RUQ	Inadequate → Poor → Good → Excellent	Normal / Abnormal
	LUQ	Inadequate → Poor → Good → Excellent	Normal / Abnormal
	Pelvic	Inadequate → Poor → Good → Excellent	Normal / Abnormal
Pipes	**IVC**	Inadequate → Poor → Good → Excellent	Normal / Abnormal
	Aorta	Inadequate → Poor → Good → Excellent	Normal / Abnormal

Abnormal clinical findings confirmed on subsequent imaging?	Yes / No / N/A

Practitioner Reflection

Provisional Diagnosis/Interpretation:

Supervisor Comments

Supervisor's Diagnosis/Interpretation:

Rapid Ultrasound for Shock & Hypotension (RUSH)

Case Study 3

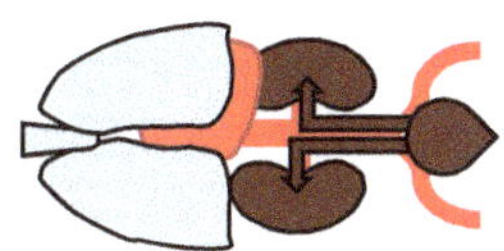

<table>
<tr><td colspan="3">Anonymised Patient Demographics</td></tr>
<tr><td>Age:</td><td></td><td>Sex:</td><td></td></tr>
<tr><td colspan="4">Indication:</td></tr>
</table>

	Views	Image Quality	Clinical finding
Pump	**Cardiac PLAX**	Inadequate → Poor → Good → Excellent	Normal / Abnormal
	Cardiac A4C	Inadequate → Poor → Good → Excellent	Normal / Abnormal
Tank	**Lung Right**	Inadequate → Poor → Good → Excellent	Normal / Abnormal
	Lung Left	Inadequate → Poor → Good → Excellent	Normal / Abnormal
	RUQ	Inadequate → Poor → Good → Excellent	Normal / Abnormal
	LUQ	Inadequate → Poor → Good → Excellent	Normal / Abnormal
	Pelvic	Inadequate → Poor → Good → Excellent	Normal / Abnormal
Pipes	**IVC**	Inadequate → Poor → Good → Excellent	Normal / Abnormal
	Aorta	Inadequate → Poor → Good → Excellent	Normal / Abnormal

Abnormal clinical findings confirmed on subsequent imaging?	Yes / No / N/A

Practitioner Reflection

Provisional Diagnosis/Interpretation:

Supervisor Comments

Supervisor's Diagnosis/Interpretation:

Rapid Ultrasound for Shock & Hypotension (RUSH)

Case Study 4

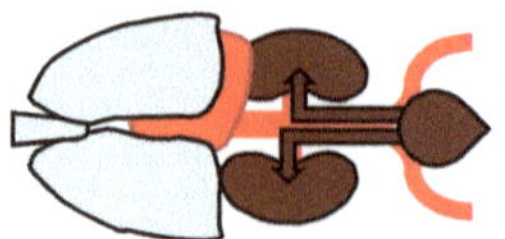

Anonymised Patient Demographics			
Age:		**Sex:**	
Indication:			

	Views	Image Quality	Clinical finding
Pump	**Cardiac PLAX**	Inadequate → Poor → Good → Excellent	Normal / Abnormal
	Cardiac A4C	Inadequate → Poor → Good → Excellent	Normal / Abnormal
Tank	**Lung Right**	Inadequate → Poor → Good → Excellent	Normal / Abnormal
	Lung Left	Inadequate → Poor → Good → Excellent	Normal / Abnormal
	RUQ	Inadequate → Poor → Good → Excellent	Normal / Abnormal
	LUQ	Inadequate → Poor → Good → Excellent	Normal / Abnormal
	Pelvic	Inadequate → Poor → Good → Excellent	Normal / Abnormal
Pipes	**IVC**	Inadequate → Poor → Good → Excellent	Normal / Abnormal
	Aorta	Inadequate → Poor → Good → Excellent	Normal / Abnormal

Abnormal clinical findings confirmed on subsequent imaging?	Yes / No / N/A

Practitioner Reflection

Provisional Diagnosis/Interpretation:

Supervisor Comments

Supervisor's Diagnosis/Interpretation:

Rapid Ultrasound for Shock & Hypotension (RUSH)

Case Study 5

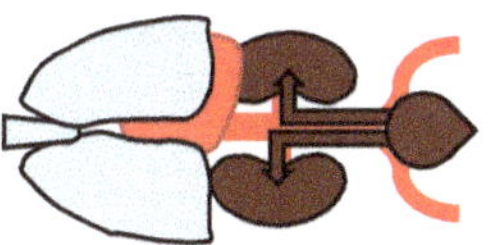

Anonymised Patient Demographics			
Age:		Sex:	
Indication:			

	Views	Image Quality	Clinical finding
Pump	**Cardiac PLAX**	Inadequate → Poor → Good → Excellent	Normal / Abnormal
	Cardiac A4C	Inadequate → Poor → Good → Excellent	Normal / Abnormal
Tank	**Lung Right**	Inadequate → Poor → Good → Excellent	Normal / Abnormal
	Lung Left	Inadequate → Poor → Good → Excellent	Normal / Abnormal
	RUQ	Inadequate → Poor → Good → Excellent	Normal / Abnormal
	LUQ	Inadequate → Poor → Good → Excellent	Normal / Abnormal
	Pelvic	Inadequate → Poor → Good → Excellent	Normal / Abnormal
Pipes	**IVC**	Inadequate → Poor → Good → Excellent	Normal / Abnormal
	Aorta	Inadequate → Poor → Good → Excellent	Normal / Abnormal

Abnormal clinical findings confirmed on subsequent imaging?	Yes / No / N/A

Practitioner Reflection

Provisional Diagnosis/Interpretation:

Supervisor Comments

Supervisor's Diagnosis/Interpretation:

Rapid DVT Protocol
Case Study 1

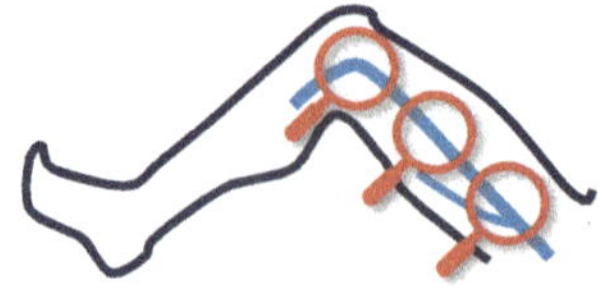

<table>
<tr><td colspan="2">Anonymised Patient Demographics</td></tr>
<tr><td>Age:</td><td>Sex:</td></tr>
<tr><td colspan="2">Indication:</td></tr>
</table>

	Fully Compressible	Occlusive Thrombus	Non-Occlusive Thrombus	Not Visualised
Common Femoral Vein Right	YES / NO	YES / NO	YES / NO	☐
Common Femoral Vein Left	YES / NO	YES / NO	YES / NO	☐
Femoral Vein Right	YES / NO	YES / NO	YES / NO	☐
Femoral Vein Left	YES / NO	YES / NO	YES / NO	☐
Popliteal Vein Right	YES / NO	YES / NO	YES / NO	☐
Popliteal Vein Left	YES / NO	YES / NO	YES / NO	☐

Practitioner Reflection

Provisional Diagnosis/Interpretation:

Supervisor Comments

Supervisor's Diagnosis/Interpretation:

Rapid DVT Protocol
Case Study 2

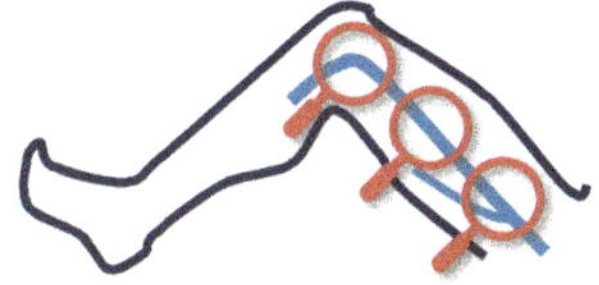

Anonymised Patient Demographics		
Age:		**Sex:**
Indication:		

	Fully Compressible	Occlusive Thrombus	Non-Occlusive Thrombus	Not Visualised
Common Femoral Vein Right	YES / NO	YES / NO	YES / NO	☐
Common Femoral Vein Left	YES / NO	YES / NO	YES / NO	☐
Femoral Vein Right	YES / NO	YES / NO	YES / NO	☐
Femoral Vein Left	YES / NO	YES / NO	YES / NO	☐
Popliteal Vein Right	YES / NO	YES / NO	YES / NO	☐
Popliteal Vein Left	YES / NO	YES / NO	YES / NO	☐

Practitioner Reflection

Provisional Diagnosis/Interpretation:

Supervisor Comments

Supervisor's Diagnosis/Interpretation:

Rapid DVT Protocol
Case Study 3

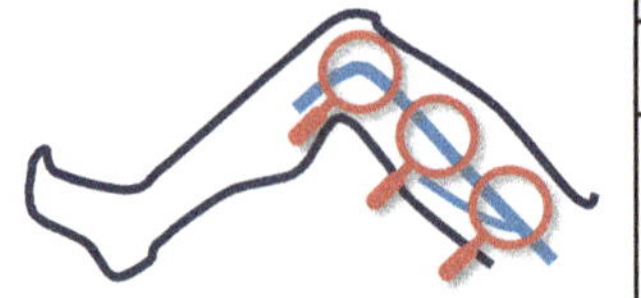

	Anonymised Patient Demographics	
Age:		Sex:
Indication:		

	Fully Compressible	Occlusive Thrombus	Non-Occlusive Thrombus	Not Visualised
Common Femoral Vein Right	YES / NO	YES / NO	YES / NO	☐
Common Femoral Vein Left	YES / NO	YES / NO	YES / NO	☐
Femoral Vein Right	YES / NO	YES / NO	YES / NO	☐
Femoral Vein Left	YES / NO	YES / NO	YES / NO	☐
Popliteal Vein Right	YES / NO	YES / NO	YES / NO	☐
Popliteal Vein Left	YES / NO	YES / NO	YES / NO	☐

Practitioner Reflection
Provisional Diagnosis/Interpretation:

Supervisor Comments
Supervisor's Diagnosis/Interpretation:

Rapid DVT Protocol
Case Study 4

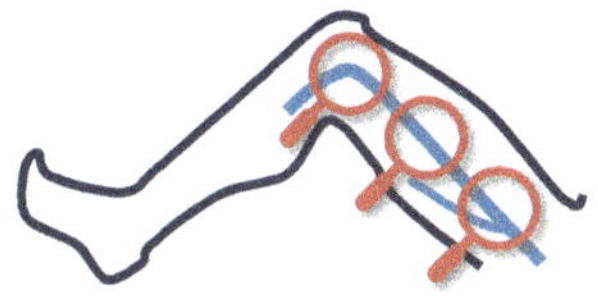

Anonymised Patient Demographics		
Age:		**Sex:**
Indication:		

	Fully Compressible	Occlusive Thrombus	Non-Occlusive Thrombus	Not Visualised
Common Femoral Vein Right	YES / NO	YES / NO	YES / NO	☐
Common Femoral Vein Left	YES / NO	YES / NO	YES / NO	☐
Femoral Vein Right	YES / NO	YES / NO	YES / NO	☐
Femoral Vein Left	YES / NO	YES / NO	YES / NO	☐
Popliteal Vein Right	YES / NO	YES / NO	YES / NO	☐
Popliteal Vein Left	YES / NO	YES / NO	YES / NO	☐

Practitioner Reflection
Provisional Diagnosis/Interpretation:

Supervisor Comments
Supervisor's Diagnosis/Interpretation:

Rapid DVT Protocol
Case Study 5

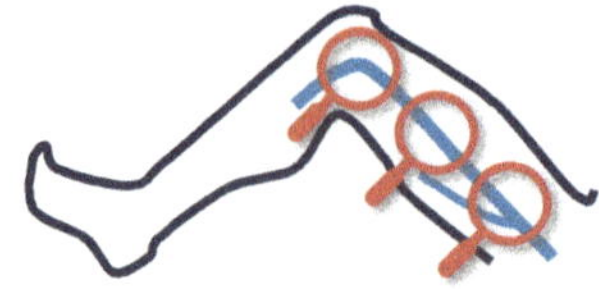

Anonymised Patient Demographics			
Age:		**Sex:**	
Indication:			

	Fully Compressible	Occlusive Thrombus	Non-Occlusive Thrombus	Not Visualised
Common Femoral Vein Right	YES / NO	YES / NO	YES / NO	☐
Common Femoral Vein Left	YES / NO	YES / NO	YES / NO	☐
Femoral Vein Right	YES / NO	YES / NO	YES / NO	☐
Femoral Vein Left	YES / NO	YES / NO	YES / NO	☐
Popliteal Vein Right	YES / NO	YES / NO	YES / NO	☐
Popliteal Vein Left	YES / NO	YES / NO	YES / NO	☐

Practitioner Reflection
Provisional Diagnosis/Interpretation:

Supervisor Comments
Supervisor's Diagnosis/Interpretation:

GENERIC REFLECTION

Case Study 1

Anonymised Patient Demographics			
Age:		**Sex:**	
Scan Type:			
Indication:			

View	Image Quality (circle)	Clinical finding (circle)
	Inadequate → Poor → Good → Excellent	Normal / Abnormal
	Inadequate → Poor → Good → Excellent	Normal / Abnormal
	Inadequate → Poor → Good → Excellent	Normal / Abnormal
	Inadequate → Poor → Good → Excellent	Normal / Abnormal
	Inadequate → Poor → Good → Excellent	Normal / Abnormal

Abnormal clinical findings confirmed on subsequent imaging?	Yes / No / N/A

Practitioner Reflection

Provisional Diagnosis/Interpretation:

Supervisor Comments

Supervisor's Diagnosis/Interpretation:

GENERIC REFLECTION

Case Study 2

Anonymised Patient Demographics			
Age:		**Sex:**	
Scan Type:			
Indication:			

View	Image Quality (circle)	Clinical finding (circle)
	Inadequate → Poor → Good → Excellent	Normal / Abnormal
	Inadequate → Poor → Good → Excellent	Normal / Abnormal
	Inadequate → Poor → Good → Excellent	Normal / Abnormal
	Inadequate → Poor → Good → Excellent	Normal / Abnormal
	Inadequate → Poor → Good → Excellent	Normal / Abnormal

Abnormal clinical findings confirmed on subsequent imaging?	Yes / No / N/A

Practitioner Reflection

Provisional Diagnosis/Interpretation:

Supervisor Comments

Supervisor's Diagnosis/Interpretation:

GENERIC REFLECTION

Case Study 3

Anonymised Patient Demographics			
Age:		**Sex:**	
Scan Type:			
Indication:			

View	Image Quality (circle)	Clinical finding (circle)
	Inadequate → Poor → Good → Excellent	Normal / Abnormal
	Inadequate → Poor → Good → Excellent	Normal / Abnormal
	Inadequate → Poor → Good → Excellent	Normal / Abnormal
	Inadequate → Poor → Good → Excellent	Normal / Abnormal
	Inadequate → Poor → Good → Excellent	Normal / Abnormal

Abnormal clinical findings confirmed on subsequent imaging?	Yes / No / N/A

Practitioner Reflection

Provisional Diagnosis/Interpretation:

Supervisor Comments

Supervisor's Diagnosis/Interpretation:

GENERIC REFLECTION

Case Study 4

Anonymised Patient Demographics			
Age:		**Sex:**	
Scan Type:			
Indication:			

View	Image Quality (circle)	Clinical finding (circle)
	Inadequate → Poor → Good → Excellent	Normal / Abnormal
	Inadequate → Poor → Good → Excellent	Normal / Abnormal
	Inadequate → Poor → Good → Excellent	Normal / Abnormal
	Inadequate → Poor → Good → Excellent	Normal / Abnormal
	Inadequate → Poor → Good → Excellent	Normal / Abnormal

Abnormal clinical findings confirmed on subsequent imaging?	Yes / No / N/A

Practitioner Reflection

Provisional Diagnosis/Interpretation:

Supervisor Comments

Supervisor's Diagnosis/Interpretation:

GENERIC REFLECTION

Case Study 5

Anonymised Patient Demographics		
Age:		**Sex:**
Scan Type:		
Indication:		

View	Image Quality (circle)	Clinical finding (circle)
	Inadequate → Poor → Good → Excellent	Normal / Abnormal
	Inadequate → Poor → Good → Excellent	Normal / Abnormal
	Inadequate → Poor → Good → Excellent	Normal / Abnormal
	Inadequate → Poor → Good → Excellent	Normal / Abnormal
	Inadequate → Poor → Good → Excellent	Normal / Abnormal

Abnormal clinical findings confirmed on subsequent imaging?	Yes / No / N/A

Practitioner Reflection

Provisional Diagnosis/Interpretation:

Supervisor Comments

Supervisor's Diagnosis/Interpretation:

The Journey to Expert

Developing competence and expertise in Point of Care Ultrasound (PoCUS) is an ongoing journey for any clinician. While a didactic course will provide a strong foundation for your professional development and progress towards expert practice, further study and exposure is required.

Multi-modal Learning

This journey of professional development should utilise multiple sources for learning, feedback and triangulation of practice. The author recommends a blend of self-directed learning, formal teaching, clinical supervision and ongoing clinical practice to ensure application of PoCUS is safe and effective for your patients.

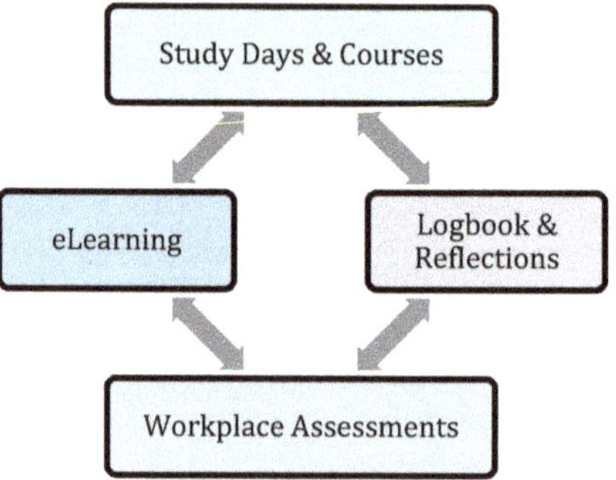

Working Towards Independent Practice

While developing your skills and competencies, it can be helpful to consider at which level of the Royal College of Emergency Medicine entrustment scale you are practising.

Point-of-Care-Ultrasound Entrustment Scale	
Level	**Descriptor**
1	Direct supervision
2 a	Indirect supervision (e.g. available in the department)
2 b	Indirect supervision (e.g. available in the building)
3	Distant supervision (e.g. on-call for advice)
4	Independent ultrasound practice

Adapted from: Royal College of Emergency Medicine. (2022). *SLO6 - Point of Care Ultrasound Competence Entrustment Scale: Guidance for Education and Training.* London.

<u>**Recommended Case Numbers**</u>

There is no consensus on recommended numbers of logged scans or reflective accounts to demonstrate proficiency. The Royal College of Emergency Medicine (2022) recommends the following for doctors undertaking training in Emergency Medicine. Other clinicians may also find this recommendation useful for their learning and development.

This logbook is designed to meet the indicative numbers detailed below.

Procedure	Reflective Accounts	Number of Logged Scans
AAA	5	25
eFAST	5	25
RUSH	5	25
ELS	5	10
Nerve Blocks	5	10
Vascular Access	5	5

Adapted from: Royal College of Emergency Medicine. (2022). *SLO6 - Point of Care Ultrasound Competence Entrustment Scale: Guidance for Education and Training.* London.

<u>**When to Utilise Ultrasound**</u>

- Diagnostic PoCUS comes into its own when it will alter treatment, facilitate more accurate triage or direct further investigations.
- If a better investigation is immediately available or PoCUS could delay meaningful interventions, <u>do not use it</u>.
- Remember that in general, PoCUS is a "rule-in" test, not a "rule-out" test.

Presentation	PoCUS Protocol
Acute abdomen	RUSH
Breathless ? Cause	Lung / IVC / Echo
Cardiac Arrest	ELS (Echo) / Lung / eFAST
Decreased GCS ? Cause	ONSD, RUSH
Shocked ? Cause	RUSH

NOTES

Ultrasound for the Generalist:
A Guide to Point of Care Imaging
(2021)
Edited by Sarb Clare and Chris Duncan

This text is the essential resource for the clinician seeking to utilise point of care ultrasound in any generalist setting.

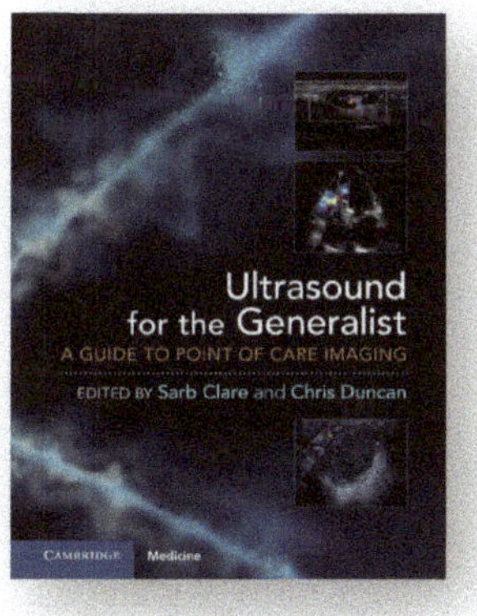

Ultrasound for the Generalist Website

The Certified Wilderness Paramedic (WP-C®) is the process to provide a globally validated measurement of Wilderness, Remote and Austere Paramedic/Practitioner knowledge. Like all other IBSC Board certifications, the WP-C® validates an individual's advanced knowledge and the critical thinking skills required for safe and competent practice in the Wilderness Paramedic/Practitioner practice domain. While a regulatory-agency issued paramedic license sets the minimum competency requirements, it is not specialty specific. The IBSC credentials provide designations for paramedic professionals who demonstrate knowledge, experience, and excellence in a specialized area of paramedicine. The WP-C® board certification examination is not reliant on any one curriculum or educational program but is based upon the unique domain of 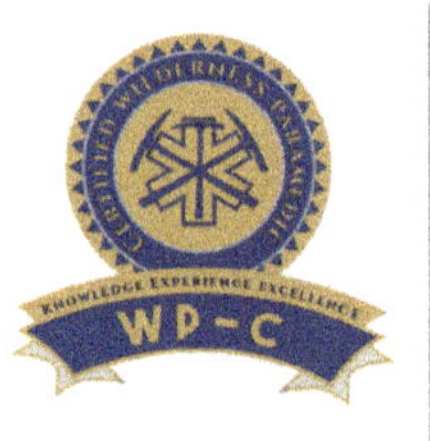 knowledge, standards, and best practices for what is already being taught and practiced in the wilderness community. Achieving board certification is the pinnacle of a specialist's lifelong commitment to demonstrating professionalism and continuous learning by becoming the best of the best.

SOCIAL MEDIA

 twitter.com/IBSCert_

 instagram.com/ibsc_certification/

 facebook.com/IBSCertifications

 linkedin.com/company/international-board-of-specialty-certifications/

International Board of Specialty Certification
300 Lockwood Road • Red Rock, TX 78662• USA
+1.770.978.4400 • help@ibsc.org

Austere and Prehospital Ultrasound©

The Austere and Prehospital Ultrasound (APUS) course is a blended online and face-to-face course developed by the College of Remote and Offshore Medicine (CoROM) to meet the demands of clinicians practising in emergency, prehospital and austere settings.

The course is accredited by the
Royal College of Surgeons of Edinburgh as of 2025.

The College of Remote and Offshore Medicine also offer a range of other CPD and higher education courses at both undergraduate and postgraduate level.
https://corom.edu.mt/

About the Author

Dr Tom E Mallinson

BSc (Hons) MBChB PGCHE DipMSK (FSEM) MRCGP (2020) MCPara MCoROM DFSEM(UK) FAWM FHEA FFRRHHEd FRGS WP-C

Paramedic, Rural GP and Prehospital Doctor, Scotland.

Senior Lecturer, College of Remote and Offshore Medicine, Malta.

Tom began his career in London, undertaking the IHCD Paramedic qualification alongside a Bachelor's Degree in Paramedic Science at the University of Hertfordshire. After working as a paramedic for the London Ambulance Service NHS Trust, he went on to attend Warwick Medical School to read Medicine. He continued his studies with postgraduate qualifications in healthcare education, wilderness medicine and primary care. Tom has published a variety of primary research and educational resources and is a member of the editorial board for the Journal of Paramedic Practice. He is a certified Wilderness Paramedic.

Author's ResearchGate Profile